ANALYSIS AND DESIGN CLASSIFICATION MODELS FOR PLANT DISEASES USING MACHINE LEARNING APPROACH

By

SANTOSH KUMAR UPADHYAY

ANALYSIS AND DESIGN OF CLASSIFICATION MODELS FOR PLANT DISEASES USING MACHINE LEARNING APPROACH

By

SANTOSH KUMAR UPADHYAY

List of Figures

List of Tables

Table of Contents

ABSTRACT

In agriculture, there are several research topics targeted at increasing production and quality while reducing costs and increasing profits. Plant development is influenced by a variety of factors, the most common of which being plant diseases. The first step in treating leaf illnesses would be to identify them. Plant leaf disease diagnosis is a field of study that examines a plant's leaf to determine whether or not it has a disease. Tracking the health and illness of a plant is extremely important to a farm's effective crop production.

The aforementioned numbers highlight the importance of early and effective disease identification in these plants, since failure or delay can result in large losses. Many studies have recently been conducted in order to address these difficulties, and this is currently a hotspot of research in the agricultural world. Paddy is the world's most important cereal crop. It is a main food for more than 50% of globe's population. Biotic and Abiotic elements such as virus, bacteria, pests, temperature, soil fertility, and precipitation influenced rice yields. Farm owners invest excessive energy and time on management of the diseases, and they guess the diseases with manual observation. The progress of technical assistance in farming has made it much easier to identify pathogens in paddy leaves automatically.

Plant diseases must be closely monitored and managed to avoid serious consequences. Disease detection is still mostly done by physical examination with the bare eyes. It is quite hard for professionals to regularly monitor big fields. Physical examination with the bare eyes might be inaccurate and ineffective. This type of procedure has been shown to be very expensive, time-consuming, and extensive.

Since image processing is an efficient tool for analyzing data, it may transform the scenario of acquiring expert advice into a cost-effective and efficient automatic decision-making system when combined with the emerging technologies like machine learning, deep learning, and IoT. Here image processing techniques are generally utilized to perform mainly 3 types of tasks (1. Image pre-processing for visual quality enhancement ,2. Image segmentation, and 3. Features Extraction). To provide computer-based disease detection system, researchers mainly focused on machine learning techniques along with digital image processing (DIP) methods. DIP techniques are utilized for quality enhancement and segmentation of input images. Quality enhancement approaches were utilized to enhance the visual characteristics of training and validation picture samples and the process of segmentation is applied to locate the infected portion in the image of plant leaves, stems, roots or fruits. In addition, relevant features are extracted from infected regions using suitable data mining and machine learning approaches. Then retrieved discriminating attributes are fed into machine learning model to perform disease recognition and classification.

Further, the introduction of deep learning (DL) approaches has made it simpler to identify agricultural diseases. DL has become a strong technology for data analytics and image processing in recent times, with promising outcomes. DL has been used in a wide range of fields, notably farming. Convolution Neural Network (CNN) is among the most widely used architectures in deep learning. Transfer learning is a novel method in deep learning that uses pre-trained architecture to train a fresh database to speed up the learning process.

In the domain of precision agriculture, automated detection and diagnosis of rice leaf infections is widely required. Rice is a common food item that is susceptible to illness. In this thesis, we have developed a total of 4 deep learning-based disease diagnosis and classification models in which 3 models are used to diagnose and classify rice diseases and one model is used to classify 9 kinds of deadly tomato diseases. In these 4 disease classification models, 2 models are based on simple fully connected Convolution neural network architecture and the remaining 2 models are transfer learning models based on pre-trained CNN architecture. For models' training and validation, we have used benchmarked rice leaf and PlantVillage datasets taken from the Kaggle platform.

In the first model, we developed a simple fully connected CNN for the detection and classification of three kinds of rice diseases (bacterial leaf blight, brown spot, and leaf smut) using leaf images. To boost performance even more, we applied the background removal technique on input images using Otsu's global thresholding technique. The results reveal that the suggested FCNN is a quick and effective solution that achieves a

99.7% accuracy on the dataset.

In second model, we introduced a method for estimating infection severity based on a two-phase image segmentation algorithm, which uses an existing plant disease dataset to generate a new dataset labeled with disease severity. The number of infected and non-infected pixels in leaf image samples is used to calculate infection severity. Next, an effective FCNN architecture is built to process this derived severity-based dataset to detect the brown spot rice disease at an early stage. The results reveal that the suggested model achieves a 99.20% accuracy.

In third model, we have used a transfer learning approach to tackle the issue of big dataset availability, and picture augmentation techniques to create variety in the visual presentation of symptoms. Using the InceptionV3 pre-trained CNN architecture along with these two techniques, an effective disease classification model is created to recognize and classify 5 types of deadly rice diseases with excellent accuracy of 100%. In fourth and last model, SqueezeNet based transfer learning model along with image augmentation technique is developed to recognize and classify the 9 kinds of deadly tomato diseases with an accuracy of 93.10%.

In last phase of this thesis, conclusion and future scope of the complete thesis work is discussed.

CHAPTER 1

INTRODUCTION

Plants are regarded as an essential source of life on the Earth. Among the almost 1.7 million varieties of living organisms, that included human beings, animals, algae, and plants, the plant is the most crucial to all remaining living organism. Human existence is dependent on plants because if plants remain, humans remain as well. Plants fulfill various requirements, including food, medicine, cloth and house. Plants serve as the foundation of the food chain in the environment. Plants also provide the basis for the majority of drugs, including Ayurvedic remedies.

A good harvest not only benefits the farmers, but it also contributes significantly to the nation's economic development. However, obtaining desired production levels is difficult due to a variety of factors such as diseases, pests, climate and many more. Keeping the utilization of the plants in mind, the identification of plant diseases becomes the most important, since right identification leads to better crops production.

Plant Illnesses are a natural element of the environment and one of the several ecological variables that serve to maintain the millions of living organisms in equilibrium with each other. Plant diseases have been recognized since the time of the first literature. Plants were harmed by illness 250 million years ago, according to fossil records. Diseases like blights, mildews and rusts, caused starvation and other significant shifts in the economies of countries since the beginning of the civilization.

A plant becomes unhealthy when it is repeatedly disrupted by certain causative factor including biological and environmental, resulting in an unusual life processes that disturbs the plant's normal development, structure, and function. Disease affects all species of plant, both cultivated and wild. Plant disease occurrence and infection severity vary seasonally, regarding the environmental circumstances, the kinds of crops cultivated, and the existence of the pathogen. Certain plant species are

1

especially vulnerable to disease outbreaks, but many others are less susceptible to them.

For thousands of years, people have thoughtfully picked and grown plants for clothing, food, shelter, beauty, fiber, and medicine. Disease is one of the deadliest hazards among several risks that must be addressed when plants are removed from their native habitat and cultivated in the fields under sometimes unfavorable conditions. Many important ornamental and crop plants are highly vulnerable to infection and would struggle to survive in the nature without humans' involvement. Planted crops are frequently more prone to infections than their wild counterparts. This is due to the fact that enormous plants of the same breed, with a similar genetic profile, are grown in close proximity, often spanning hundreds of Kilo-metre square.

1.1 Crop Disease an Overview

In today's globe, the farming land is not only a source of food, but also contributes a lot in economy. Indian GDP is highly dependent on the farming and its product. The presence of insects or other infections is the leading cause of agricultural yield loss; thus, the danger of yield losses may be decreased by offering a disease detection solution in the agriculture [1].

Expert eye observation was used in the past to detect plant diseases. However, they were time demanding and involved a considerable danger of personal perception.

Plant disease identification and classification is a long-standing issue that concerns the farming industry. Various research techniques are applied to accurately recognize and classify crop disease in a variety of plants. These range from traditional expert on-field examination to the application of image processing methods, as well as the more contemporary application of ML and DL algorithms. However, due to exorbitant costs in some cases and a lack of resilience in others, the benefits of these procedures are not completely leveraged. Against these odds, transfer learning and deep learning approaches perform admirably, and the current effort employs these techniques to accurately identify and categorise plant illness.

2

1.2 Statement of Problem

Plant diseases are a worldwide hazard to feed a growing population, it may also be devastating for small-scale farmers whose lives are dependent on crops production. Small-scale farmers produce greater than 80 percent of crops yields in developing countries(UNEP, 2013), and more than 50% yield reduction is observed due to plant diseases and pests [2]. Moreover, small farming families belong to the class of the majority of starving people (Fifty percent) [3], these small-scale farmers are always sensitive to pathogen-related food supply disruptions.

In the age of environmental changes around the world plant diseases have become a problem because they can reduce the amount of production and quality of agricultural goods significantly. Automatic-detection of crop illnesses is a key research domain because it might help in monitoring the huge fields of crops and, as a result, recognize disease signs as-soon-as they occur on plant leaves. Precise recognition and diagnosis of crop diseases is essential for food security and the control of the spread of exotic pathogens/pests This allows image-based automated evaluation, control systems, and robot-guiding using machine-vision. Visual recognition, on the other hand, is time-consuming, inaccurate, and limited to narrow crop fields. Though improvements have been achieved in all dimensions of plant disease detection; boosting accuracy, specificity, sensitivity and efficiency have remained a crucial issue that should be addressed. The suggested system is an effective solution for detecting and classifying plant leaf diseases automatically and accurately. We proposed an approach to capture the diseases at initial stage.

1.3 Motivation

Visual investigation by naked eyes is still the primary technique of disease diagnosis in villages of developing countries [4]. These traditional methods require skilled monitoring on a regular basis. Many of the farmers detect the plant diseases manually on self-experience basis. Generally, this self-investigation does not capture initial symptoms of the infection at early stage of diseases which gives chance to the

3

pathogens to spread out in the whole crop fields. Many times, this visual inspection fails to recognize the diseases accurately. Some aware farmers feel it appropriate to take expert advice to identify the disease. Therefore, farmers in remote areas need to plan a long journey to see a plant pathologist, that is both expensive and time-taking [5,6]. Certainly, laboratory-based illness detection is more precise. But it leads to diagnosis delays. Late diagnosis causes a reduction in crop yields. Hence, automated and accurate disease identification in plants is very important to ensure better quantity and quality of crops.

1.4 Plant Diseases and its types

Plant diseases are broadly classified into 2 types: pathogenic and non- pathogenic.

1.4.1 Pathogenic Disease

Pathogenic diseases are also known as parasitic or infectious diseases. Pathogenic illnesses are caused by infectious microorganisms. This type of diseases spread very fast due to pathogen's ability of being multiply at fast rate. Major causing organisms of this sort of illnesses are Bacteria, fungus, and virus. Figure 1.1 depicts the types of pathogenic diseases.

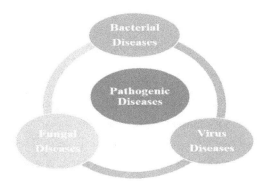

Figure 1.1 Types of Pathogenic Diseases

4

1) Bacterial Diseases

Bacterial leaf spot is a common name for a bacterial illness. In order for the bacteria to cause an illness in a plant, the bacteria first penetrate and multiply in the tissue of plant. Most bacteria cause only one significant symptom, while some cause a variety or mix of symptoms. In general, determining if a plant is infected with a bacterial infection is not hard; however, identifying the pathogenic organism at the initial level necessitates separation and identification of the microorganism using a variety of laboratory procedures. Moisture and temperature have a big impact on bacterial illnesses. Usually, a small temperature difference decides whether or not a bacterial illness will emerge. In several situations, moisture in the form of a water layer on leaves and stems surfaces is one of the main reasons for developing an infection. It begins as tiny, yellow-green spots on new leaves that are distorted and curled, or as greasy-looking lesions with water-soaked and dark appearance on older leaves and stems. The majority of foliage parasites travel from one infected plant to other by dust, rain, and wind. Following are some commons symptoms caused by bacteria:

a) Necrosis

b) Vascular wilt

c) Tumours

d) Soft rot

2) Fungal Diseases

Fungi are responsible for the bulk of contagious plant infections, accounts for nearly two-thirds. All economically significant crops appear to be affected by fungus; in many cases, many fungi may spread infection in a single species of plants. Usually, widespread or local necrosis is caused by a fungal disease. It can either slow down the usual development or cause extreme aberrant development in a part or the whole plant. Fungi propagate mostly by spores, which are abundant. Dust, water, wind

5

streams, birds, insects, and the remnants of diseased plants can all carry and spread the infection. Following are some commons symptoms caused by fungi:

a) The majority of flower, fruit, and leaf spots

b) All true and white rusts, sooty moulds, mildew, smuts, anthracnoses, leaf curls, and needle casts

c) blights

d)cankers

e) Shoot, bud and leaf galls

d) wilts

e) Scabs, wood, fruit, root, and stem rots and many more

3) Virus Diseases

They can only grow or reproduce within a live cell of a specific host. A single species of plants can be infected by multiple distinct viruses. Virus infection causes major illness in essential food plants like palm, sugarcane, rice, corn, oats, wheat, tomato, potato, sugar beet, orange, and peach. Infections are often more severe in crops cultivated asexually—that is, through sprouts, cut divisions, and cuttings, in comparison of crops cultivated sexually by using seeds. Following are some commons symptoms caused by viruses:

a) Dwarfing of whole plants or stems, leaves

b) Necrosis (internal death, drooping or wilting, streaks, circular spots, and

leaf spots)

c) Malformations (proliferation, rosetting, deformation of flowers and leaves)

d) Variation in color (vein clearing, yellow mottling, yellowing)

1.4.2 Non-pathogenic Disease

Non-pathogenic diseases are also known as non-parasitic or non- infectious diseases. These types of illnesses, which might appear abruptly, are created by a lack of availability, a deficiency, an inappropriate balance, or an excess of climatic and soil parameters. Non-pathogenic illnesses in plants can emerge as a result of;

a) Mechanical injuries caused by animals or human being,

b) Genetic defects in seeds

c)Air pollution in environment

d) Toxic chemicals

e) Variations in climatic factors (temperature, moisture, humidity, rain etc.)

f) changes in soil parameters (organic matter, texture, soil humidity, soil pH, etc.), and so on.

1.5 Samples of Pathogenic plant diseases

This part quickly covers many categories of crop illnesses that are very common in several crops. Brief description along with sample images of some of the most common illnesses found in certain crops are presented here.

1.5.1 Rice diseases

Following are some common plant diseases found in rice crops.

1) Brown spot: Brown spot is a deadly infection caused by fungal disease. The spikelets, coleoptile, glumes, leaves, panicle branches, and leaf sheath are all infected with this infection. The most visible injury that appears on the leaves is multiple large lesions that can destroy the entire leaf. When a seed becomes infected, it produces empty grains or discolored or spotted seeds.

2) Bacterial leaf blight: It mostly damages the plant's leaves. This condition manifests as elongated patches of few inches long. Lesions on the entire leaf may appear as the illness advances. The white color spots become yellow as the infection of bacteria increases. This illness is transmitted mostly by wind stream and water. This illness is caused by bacterial pathogen Xanthomonas oryzae.

3) Leaf smut: Crop's leaves are mostly targeted and damaged in this disease. This infection appears as angular black spot that is slightly elevated. Other symptoms include dull patches with reddish-brown edges visible on the leaves. This illness is caused by a fungal pathogen known as Entyloma oryzae. Infected plant waste mixed in the soil and water spreads this virus. This virus is also transmitted by airborne spores.

4) Leaf blast: The fungal organism Magnaporthe oryzae causes leaf blast. It harms the components of a rice plant that lies above the soil, including the leaf sheath, panicle sections, neck, node leaf, collar, and the leaf. Lesions that are spindle or oval shaped with brown border appear on the affected parts of the plant.

5) Sheath blight: It causes appearance of lesions on the leaves. It leads generation of hollow grains. Water-soaked to greenish grey color patches are found on infected leaves in initial infection. As the disease spreads, lesion's color become gray. The causal organism is fungal pathogen named as Rhizoctonia solani.

6) Tungro: The virus that causes paddy tungro infection is a combination of 2 viruses (RTSV and RTBV) carried by leafhoppers. Partially filled or even empty seeds in severe cases, fewer tillers, slower growth, and darker lesions are the symptoms appeared on the leaf. The darkening begins at the tip of the leaves and extends to the blade.

7) "Leaf-scald": It is a fungal-infection produced by "Microdochium-oryzae" that causes scalded leaves. The pathogen of this infection, which damages seedlings, panicles, and leaves is seed-borne and persists across the plants on contaminated seed. The infection often appears on mature leaves.

1.5.2 Tomato Diseases

Following are some common plant diseases found in tomato crops.

1) Target spot: Target spot is a fungal-disease that damages the stems, fruits, and leaves of plants. This infection is very common in plants namely papaya, tomato, legumes, and cucumber. Causing pathogen of the target spot is Corynesporacassiicola. In the early- stage it starts with tiny irregular-shaped spots on old leaves. Later these spots become enlarged (up to 10 mm) with the appearance of concentric brown spots. Margins of these spots are observed as yellow.

2) Tomato Mosaic Virus: This deadly disease is caused by Tomato mosaic virus. Mosaic infection mainly damages the stems and leaves of the plants. Symptoms include a dark and light green mottled appearance on the leaves. The damaged plant is pale green, undersized, and wiry in appearance.

3) Tomato yellow leaf curl virus: The upward curling and yellowing of the leaves, which can often seem crumpled, are the most typical symptoms of the condition. Plants that have been affected seem undersized, pale, and bushy in appearance. "Tomato yellow leaf curl" virus is the causal organism of this infection.

4) Bacterial Spot: This is a Bacterial infection. In Bacterial spots dark, tiny, ring-to-irregular-shaped spots appear on the leaves, that may be encircled by a yellow halo. The infections usually appear on the leaf tips and margins, and lesions can be enlarged up to 3-5 mm in diameter. The leaves of infected plants may seem burned. The causal organism is Xanthomonas campestris pv. Vesicatoria.

5) Early Blight: Early-Blight is a fungal-infection that is caused by a pathogen namely Alternaria-solani. Symptoms appear as tiny brown spots on older and lower leaves that grow to about 0.25- 0.50 inches in diameter in form of a concentric circle. In advance cases, whole leaves become yellow and die. This infection affects fruits, leaves, stems, and the upper part of plants.

6) Late Blight: Late blight manifests itself as a water-soaked irregular shape with a small halo or circle around the lesions on older leaves. This infection appears with grey spots on the lower and older leaves. In advance cases, the whole plant (including leaves, fruits, and stems) is infected which may lead to total crops failure. Late Blight is a fungal infection that is caused by the organism Phytophthora infestans.

7) Tomato Leaf Mold: The lesions begin as pale green tiny dots on the top sides of the leaves which turn into yellowish spots. In case of advanced infection, spots merge and become bright yellow. Diseased leaves curl and die. This is a fungal infection that is caused by the organism Passalora fulva.

8) Septoria Leaf Spot: On leaves, there are tiny, circular to irregular shaped spots with a grey color dot at the center and a black margin. Spots commonly begin on lower and older leaves and progress upwards. This is a fungal infection caused by the organism Septoria lycopersici.

9) Two-spotted spider mite: Mite feeding produces leaf bronzing or yellowing at first. The upper leaf sides are generally mottled or speckled, and the progression of this injury causes the leaves to drop. This disease is caused by the two-spotted spider mite (*Tetranychusurticae).*

1.5.3 Cucumber Diseases

Following are some common plant diseases found in cucumber crops.

1) Angular leaf spot: It is a dangerous infection of the cucumber crops that causes lower yields and lower quality fruits. You may initially observe the sickness during hot weather followed by rain. This disease is treated using a mix of fungicides, and excellent garden cleanliness. This is a bacterial infection. Causal organism of this disease is Pseudomonas syringae.

2) Downy mildew: Pseudoperonospora cubensis is a causal fungal pathogen of this disease. It is an obligatory parasite that requires alive cucurbit plants to thrive and survive. The fungus downy mildew typically affects the leaf, leading in reduced photosynthesis. This disease causes infection in cucumber, melons, pumpkins, squash, and gourds.

3) Powdery mildew: It is a fungal infection that appears as a grey or white powder on plant leaves, leading the leaves to distort and die. Powdery mildew is caused by the pathogen Podosphaera xanthii.

1.5.4 Wheat Diseases

1)Loose smut: It is a seed-borne disease that infects Loose Smut by wind-borne spores during flowering. The virus lies latent inside the apparently healthy-looking seed, but plants developed from these seeds have diseased inflorescence.

2) Stripe rust: It appears in beginning of spring, when humidity is high and temperatures are low. The main signs are orange-yellow-colored narrow stripes on the glumes, awns, sheaths, and leaves. Stripe-rust is caused by the fungus Puccinia-striiformis.

3) Powdery mildew: Powdery mildew appears as the powdery patches of the white colour on the stem and upper surface of leaf. On the floral sections, stem, sheath, and leaf, greyish white powdery development occurs. Powdery growth develops into a black patch, causing the leaves and other components to dry out.

4) Brown rust: The upper leaf blades are the most susceptible parts for infection, although awns, glumes, and sheaths, can also get infected and show symptoms. The pustules are slightly elliptical or round, narrower than lesions of the stem rust. Brown rust is also known as leaf rust. This fungal disease is caused by Puccinia triticina.

5) Yellow rust: Mostly found on the leaves, but also on the stem and the leaf sheaths. At a preliminary phase of crop, bright yellow pustules (Uredia) emerge on the leaves, and the pustules are grouped as stripes. The stripes range in colour from yellow to orange yellow. Puccinia striiformis is the causal fungus of this disease.

1.5.5 Potato Diseases

1) Bacterial wilt: This disease also harms crops like egg plant, chilli, tobacco, tomato, and various weed species. All portions of affected plants exhibit signs of bacterial wilt disease. Infection spreads from the tips of the leaf to all portions of the plant. The leaf bases become yellow, and the plant wilts and dies. This bacterial disease is caused by pathogen; Ralstonia solanacearum.

2) Late Blight: This illness causes damage to the tubers, stems, and leaves. Infected leaf appears scalded, blistered, then dry and die. When foliage dries out, they turn black or brown. Causal pathogen is fungus-like microorganism named as Phytophthora infestans.

3) Early Blight: This is a prevalent potato disease that appears on the leaves at any phase of growth and creates distinctive blight and leaf spots. Usually, illness symptoms appear at the tuber bulging phase and progress to harvest. Early blight appears on older leaves as tiny, dark spots. Lesions grow in size until they are 1/4 inch or more in diameter, at which point bull's eye patterned concentric circles can be observed in the middle of the infected region. This fungal disease is caused by Alternaria solani.

4) Black Scurf: Infection invade plant tissue and induce stolon blindness, resulting in decreased tuber growth. Tubers infected by this disease cause generation of black scurf; however, this is primarily decorative in nature, it does not reduce the yields. This fungal infection is caused by pathogen; Rhizoctonia solani.

1.6 Image based plant Diseases Detection and Classification

Plant illnesses are a crucial issue in farming that reduces the eminence and quantity of the plant yields. The detection and classification models are a typical strategy applied in farming to diagnose the crop diseases.

Disease recognition is a process of determining whether a specific disease present in the plant or not. Image processing techniques are frequently used to detect illness and also to estimate its severity. Classification techniques may be viewed as variations of detection systems, however, instead of attempting to identify only one particular illness among several diseases, classification methods detect and name the diseases harming the plant. Usually, classification techniques follow a segmentation and features extraction unit. The segmentation process identifies interested area in the input sample and the feature extraction technique obtains relevant features from the segmented image. In plant disease detection and classification system, generally images of leaf or stem, or fruit are acquired from the plant and use as input image for the disease detection system. These extracted features are then fed into some form of classifier. We have done a deep survey on plant disease recognition and classification systems. Different systems used different approaches. We have organised these approaches as shown in Figure 1.2.

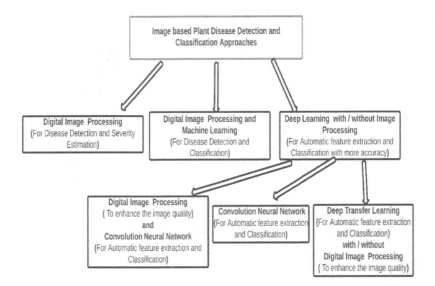

Figure 1.2 Plant disease recognition approaches based on leaf images

These approaches can be classified in 5 parts.

1) DIP (To recognize the diseases and to estimate the disease severity)

2) DIP with ML approach (To classify and recognize the diseases)

3) Deep CNN (To classify the diseases by automatically extracting the features)

4) DIP (To enhance the image quality) and Convolution Neural Network (To classify the diseases by automatically extracting the features)

5) Deep Transfer Learning (For Automatic feature extraction and Classification) with / without Digital Image Processing (To improve the image visual characteristics)

We have arranged and discussed these approaches in 4 broad categories in following subsections 1.6.1, 1.6.2, 1.6.3, and 1.6.4. We have combined 3rd and 4th approaches in one category named as "Automatic feature extraction and classification with Deep learning". First approach is discussed in subsection 1.6.1 under topic "plant disease detection using image processing". Second approach is discussed in subsection 1.6.2 under topic "Disease Detection and classification using image processing and machine learning". 3rd and 4th techniques are discussed in subsection 1.6.3 under topic "Automatic feature extraction and classification with Deep learning (Convolution Neural Network)". Furthermore, fifth approach is illustrated in subsection 1.6.4 under topic "Use of transfer learning for efficient and effective disease detection and classification result".

1.6.1 Detection of Plant Diseases using Image Processing

Researchers leverage spectroscopy and image processing techniques to remove the problems associated with manual plant disease detection methods. In our study, we explore contribution of image-processing techniques in domain of plant-disease-detection. We have not covered spectroscopy technique here. In this section, plant disease detection and/or severity estimation process using digital image processing is discussed. The fundamental steps required for "disease detection" using DIP is shown in Figure 1.3.

The process of detecting plant diseases using DIP techniques is divided into the following steps:

1) Image capture: This is very first step in DIP technique. In this process, relevant image (s) is/are collected either directly from crop fields or from well-known datasets. Generally, images of roots, or stems, or branches, or leaves, or fruits are captured from interested plant. In our research, we have utilized leaves images of the plant to conduct the experiments.

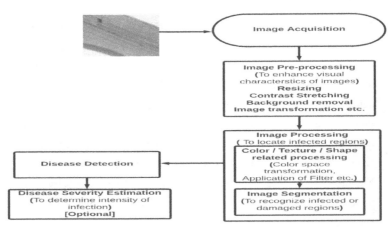

Figure 1.3 Fundamental steps required for disease detection using DIP

2) Image pre-processing: This step is required to get quality images for further processing. In this process visual appearance and characteristics are improved using several image-processing operations. The resizing operation is used to speed up the image processing computation by reducing the size of images. Contrast stretching operation (CLAHE, LAHE etc.) can be used to improve visual appearance of images. Similarly, back ground removal procedures can be carried out to get interested object from input image [7]. Image transformation may be rotation, scaling, translation, and reflection of images. Any image transformation operation can be used as per research requirement. Many more such image processing operations are available, that may be used as image pre-processing operation.

15

3) Image Processing: These are main computations performed on images to solve the research problems. These operations are applied on pre-processed images to get better results. Color, texture and morphological characteristics of images are analysed in this module. Image segmentation is applied to check abnormality in leaf, stem or fruit images. These image segmentation techniques are based on color/shape/texture.

4) Disease detection and/or Severity Estimation: Once infected regions are located successfully in leaf or fruit using segmentation technique, then disease severity is computed by computing area of infected regions.

1.6.2 Disease Recognition and Classification using DIP and ML together

Image processing approaches are intended to enhance agricultural productivity by aiding in agricultural field monitoring. Computer vision, in conjunction with soft computing/ML techniques, has been used in various plant pathology studies ("Sabrol and Kumar 2015; Singh et al. 2015a, b") [8,9,10]. The process of detecting crop illnesses using DIP and ML techniques is divided into the following modules: picture capture, image pre-processing, image segmentation, feature extraction, and identification or classification. A fundamental diagram of this approach is depicted in Figure 1.4.

Adequate training of a classification model on acquired images is needed for accurate identification; First of all, images of interesting parts like stems, roots, leaves, and fruits are acquired from the plants. After image acquisition, numerous pre-processing operations such as smoothening, rotation, scaling, contrast stretching, transformation, etc., are utilized on acquired input images as needed to get cleaned and quality images. Segmentation is then implemented to achieve the regions of interest from the diseased part of plants (leaves/stems/fruits images). Furthermore, the characterising attributes are obtained from the infected region and these features are utilised to provide the training to the classification model. Classification model is designed using ML methods ("SVM, decision tree, Naïve bayes classifier, ANN, etc").

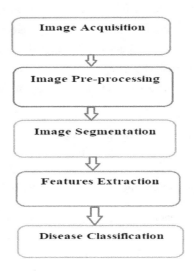

Figure 1.4 Fundamental steps of plant disease classification using ML techniques
[7]

During the validation step, the trained model determines whether the illness seen in the test picture is healthy or infected. Prior to this, the test pictures pass through all of the same stages as the train pictures to achieve significant characteristics from test images.

1.6.3 Classification by Automatically extracting the features with Deep learning (CNN)

In the fields of "image-processing and computer-vision", the attention has recently shifted to deep learning (DL) ("Szegedy et al. 2015, LeCun et al., 2015; Cruz et al. 2017") [11,12,13]. DL has demonstrated impressive performances in fields including object recognition, object identification [14], biological picture categorization [15,16], and speech recognition [17]. To use deep neural network capabilities to detect and classify crop diseases, the CNN model has been used most frequently. CNN is

17

capable of performing both tasks feature extraction and classification in one unit. Deep learning is a new technique for extracting features from leaf photos automatically. Convolution neural network (CNN) has been a growing topic for picture categorization due to its ability to extract features automatically. It is able to tackle large data without the need for picture pre-processing. A systematic approach of "plant disease detection and classification" using Deep CNN is depicted in Figure 1.5.

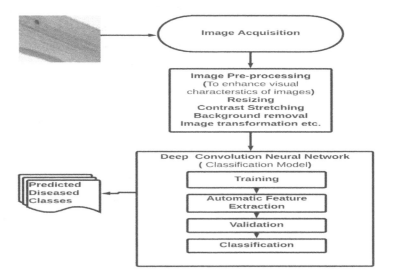

Figure 1.5 "Plant disease detection and classification" using Deep CNN

The initial stage in every DIP program is image-acquisition. The goal of image capture is to acquire pictures of the plant's sick parts. The photos are obtained either from a benchmarked dataset or directly from the agricultural field in this stage. The photographs collected are used as a train and test datasets. Image pre-processing is optional, but many researchers have used DIP concepts to improve the image quality for better classification results [7]. To sanitize the dataset, image preprocessing is performed. Image preprocessing entails a variety of activities that are carried out

18

according to the study requirements. Finally, the CNN model is developed to extract the most relevant features map and to characterize the plant diseases.

1.6.4 Use of transfer learning for efficient and effective disease detection and classification result

For the categorization of images, recently, many researchers attract towards transfer learning technique due to its ability to learn the relevant features correctly from the small available data set. Agriculture sector has also not remained untouched by it. Transfer learning not only saves the time of learning, but also gives promising classification accuracy in the fields of image recognition and classification.

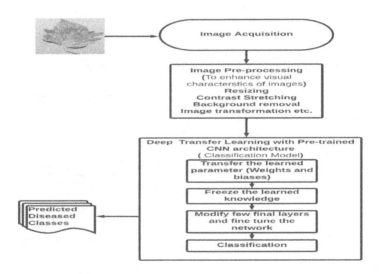

Figure 1.6 Plant illness recognition and classification using TL

The fundamental benefit of adopting TL is that, rather than beginning the learning from fresh, the model utilized the learned patterns of already solved tasks while tackling a similar nature task. As a result, the classifier may make use of prior knowledge rather than having to start from zero. Transfer learning is commonly used in image classification by the application of pre-trained networks. A pre-trained

19

model is one that has been trained on a big dataset. These pre-trained networks with the concept of transfer learning are used to tackle a problem that is comparable to the one, that has already been solved. Most frequently used pre-trained models are mobile net, VGG, Inception v3, DenseNet169, Squeeze net, ResNet50, InceptionResNet v1, InceptionResNet v2, Googlenet,etc. Generally, deep CNN architectures are pre-trained on a large Imagenet dataset [18] before applying transfer learning. Learned weights and biases of pretrained network are utilized to design a DL model for a specific task (disease detection with specific image samples). Final few layers of the pre-trained classifier are modified to make it compatible for the specific task. Finally fine tuning is performed to tune the training parameters for disease classification. A "systematic approach of plant disease detection and classification" using transfer learning is shown in Figure 1.6.

1.7 Thesis Outlines

This Thesis comprise of the following chapters:

Chapter 2 In this chapter complete Literature review, research gaps and research objectives are discussed.

Chapter 3 This chapter discusses dataset, methods and result analysis of proposed Deep CNN architecture-based Rice plant leaf disease diagnosis model.

Chapter 4 This chapter discusses dataset, methods and result analysis of proposed Deep CNN architecture-based ESBS diseases diagnosis Model for Paddy crop.

Chapter 5 This chapter discusses dataset, methods and result analysis of proposed transfer learning-based rice disease diagnosis model with small dataset and complex image background.

Chapter 6 This chapter discusses dataset, methods and result analysis of proposed transfer learning-based tomato disease diagnosis model.

Chapter 7 In this chapter conclusion of the complete thesis work is discussed.

CHAPTER 2

LITERATURE REVIEW

The relevant studies related to plant disease diagnosis and classification are included in this chapter to identify unexplored areas that could be further explored. This chapter is divided into 3 sections; first section presents review of existing methods; second section presents gap identification and third section discusses the research objectives.

2.1 Review of Existing Methods

During the 1990s, researchers and agricultural scientists started to focus their attention on computer-based solutions for disease detection and classification in plants. We have included such computer-based solutions from several peer reviewed academic journals and academic conferences in literature review.

2.1.1 Related to Plant Disease recognition using DIP techniques

In a variety of applications and domains, image-processing has shown to be an efficient-method for examining and solving related problems. From the farmers' perspective, factors such as yield, disease, and product quality were essential criteria in the agriculture industry. For a long period of time, farmers seek expert advice for solutions to agricultural problems.

Expert counsel is not always feasible, and maximum times the expert's availability and services take time. When compared to previous manual approaches, the image processing analysis for agricultural challenges (plant identification, yields prediction, fruit sorting, crop disease recognition, etc.) has proven to be more accurate and more efficient.

In this subsection, I have discussed a literature survey on various methods and approaches, which are suggested by different researchers in different years for plant leaf disease detection using image processing techniques.

In 2009, N. N. Kurniawatti et al. (2019) [19] introduced a DIP-based technique for rice disease identification and categorization. The primary goal of the present study was to create a prototype model for detecting rice illnesses such as "narrow brown-spot disease (NBSD), brown-spot disease (BSD), and blast disease (BD)". The focus of this work was to obtain rice characteristics from offline picture samples. In proposed approach, image capture was followed by automated thresholding based on the Otsu technique and local entropy threshold to transform RGB pictures into binary images. The noise was removed using a morphological algorithm namely the region filling approach. Then, from rice leaves pictures, image attributes such as damaged rice leave color, spot color, border color, and kind of lesion were retrieved. As a result of using the production rule approach, rice illnesses may be identified with an accuracy rate of 94.7 percent. This strategy has a lot of potentials to be useful. In this procedure, the Otsu threshold is utilized to detect illness spots, and the median filter was applied to eliminate any unneeded lesions.

In 2008, The approach of image pre-processing for identifying the illness lesions was presented by Ying et al. (2008) [20]. They have taken image samples of cucumber downy mildew, powdery mildew, and speckle to conduct the experiments. The impact of 2 filters, a median filter and a simple filter was studied in the suggested work. Authors ultimately picked the median filter to effectively remove noise disturbances. The median filter was utilized in this article to smooth the digital pictures and to get quality image. Interested leaf section was separated from complex background using 2-apex technique. Snake model and edge detection technique were experimented to locate lesions in diseased leaves. Snake model has given better result. The thresholding approach was applied to turn the filtered picture into a black and white image, and the infected lesions were then discovered employing the edge detection method.

In 2010, Zhang et al. (2010) [21] presented the results of establishing image processing algorithms to identify rust severity from multi-spectral pictures in

22

their work. They have applied 2 methods namely threshold setting and centroid locating to recognize rust severity. In first experiment, "sick regions were separated from leaf image by developing a rapid manual threshold-setting approach based on the Hue Saturation Intensity color space". They have determined the ratio of diseased region and the rust color index and used them as disease detection parameters to estimate the rust severity. In second experiment, centroid locating approach was developed. In centroid locating approach, firstly leaf color distribution map was determined then centroid of this distribution was analyzed to identify rust. Authors have experimented their method on 32 leaf image samples of soybean plant and it was observed that the threshold-setting-method was capable to identify rust-severity in controlled environment, while the centroid locating approach was capable to identify rest severity in real crop field environment.

Patil et al. (2011) [22] introduced an illness recognition technique based on disease severity calculation for sugar plants. They have applied thresholding segmentation techniques on plant leaves to get infected portions. These segmentations were done in 2-phases. In the first-phase, the leaf region was identified in the input image using simple thresholding. In the second phase, infected regions were identified using triangle thresholding. Finally, "diseases severity was determined by calculating the ratio of lesion area and leaf area". The algorithm's accuracy is determined by calculating the percentage difference of standard and experimented lesion area. The standard area of lesions was determined using standard shape like rectangle, square, circle and triangle using a paintbrush tool. Accuracy in percentage was computed by subtracting percentage difference of standard and experimented lesion area from 100. The average accuracy of suggested strategy was recorded as 98.60%.

In 2012, Piyush Chaudhary et al. (2012) [23] developed an automatic technique to detect infected lesion on the leaves of crop using DIP techniques. They have analysed and compared the cons and pros of different color space (HSI, YCbCr, CIELAB) used in disease detection. Authors have illustrated that CIELAB color space was very effective to remove the noises that was induced in leaf images due to leaf vein and

23

camera flash. Median filter was applied on leaf images to smooth the images. Finally, Otsu's-thresholding approach was used to segment the infected spot from leaf images.

Naikwad, S. and Amoda, N. (2013) [24] proposed a histogram matching technique to recognize plant disease. Color features and edge-detection techniques was used to match the histogram of the diseased portion in the leaf. Features were extracted using "Color Co-occurrence Method (CCM) and texture analysis". "Spatial Gray-level Dependence Matrices" were used to develop CCM. The suggested method can achieve better results with advanced color features and large datasets.

Dhaygude et al. (2013) [25] presented a plant disease detection technique consisting of four steps. This technique is based on image-segmentation and the color co-occurrence Method. In the first step, the input RGB image was converted into HSV color format. Here HSV image was utilized for a color descriptor. In the next step, green color pixels were removed and masked using a threshold value. In this step, diseased portions were achieved by removing green pixels from the leaf. In the third step, equal-sized patches were segmented from the diseased regions. Then useful patches were chosen which contains more than 50% information. Finally, in the last step, texture analysis was performed on useful segments using color co-occurance matrix to recognize the plant diseases.

Particle Swarm Optimization (PSO) is a new image segmentation technique proposed by Muthukannan and Latha (2015) [26]. PSO is a self-regulating, efficient unsupervised technique for better segmentation and feature extraction. HFE method was used to extract the relevant features. There were 3 components in this method in which one was analyzing the texture features and the other 2 components were analyzing shape and color features, respectively. The co-occurrence grey level matrices of several leaves were then used to calculate the hybrid characteristic coefficients. The suggested approach was validated on several photos of infected leaves, and the results were promising. According to the findings, the HFE strategy helped in disease classification by improving the accuracy of the classification and reducing false classification. Finally, the suggested HFE technique might be useful for improved classification of a variety of diseases found in plant leaves.

Rishi and Gill (2015) [27] discussed image processing algorithms for identifying and classifying crop diseases. They talked about how important picture compression is for disease detection. The authors investigated and examined the importance of Otsu's thresholding method for segmentation, the K-means clustering for noise removal, and image cropping in the recognition of diseases.

Zhang et al. (2017) [28] proposed a new illness recognition approach for cucumber plants that comprises three cascaded processes: K-means segmentation to segment infected leaf pictures, collecting "shape and color" characteristics from infected regions, and sparse representation (SR) for categorizing infected leaf images. The classification in the SR space may significantly cut computational costs and increase detection rate, which is a great benefit of this technique. This method is able to detect 7 most frequent leaf diseases found in cucumber plants with an overall detection accuracy of 85.7%.

Singh and Misra (2017) [29] applied soft computing to segment the diseased region in plant leaf. This study proposed a method for picture segmentation, which was used to recognize and categorize the diseases found in plant leaves automatically. It also included an overview of several disease categorization systems that may be utilized to detect leaf diseases. The genetic algorithm is used to do "image segmentation", which is an important part of "disease detection" in plant leaf disease.

As per the above discussion, we have seen that DIP techniques for identifying crop diseases and determining the severity of crop diseases are efficient, accurate, and convenient. It will assist farmers in determining the precise amount of insecticide needed to apply, lowering the disease management costs and reducing the environmental pollution. Traditional approach's human-induced mistakes and subjectivity are no longer an issue. But image processing alone is not able to build a smart system for disease detection and classification, which can learn characterizing features from the input data. An automatic\intelligent\smart disease recognition and classification model can be built by combining DIP operations with ML and/or DL techniques. In the next subsection, we have surveyed various techniques that used DIP operations in combination with ML techniques to diagnose leaf illness found in various plants.

2.1.2 Related to Plant Disease Recognition and Classification using ML along with DIP Techniques

In this subsection, we have discussed a "literature review" on various techniques and approaches, which were suggested by different researchers in different years for plant leaf disease diagnosis and categorization using various DIP techniques in combination with ML approaches. In these systems, lesions identification was done by DIP techniques and disease classification was performed by ML models. Here image processing techniques are utilized in following order:

1. To enhance visual characteristics of images
2. To segment the interested region from input image
3. To retrieve the significant visual features (Texture, morphological, and color features) from segmented regions.

While ML techniques are utilized to perform classification task.

In 1999, Sasakoi et al. (1999) [30] determined shape and spectral reflection features by using genetic algorithms to diagnose the infections in the plant. In this paper, automated identification method for cucumber anthracnose was suggested by the authors. The impact of optical filtering on illness identification is based on distinct spectral reflection properties. To diagnose disorders, they employed a genetic algorithm to build identification factors based on 2 angles of spectral reflection and attributes of the shapes of sample images. Conventional computer vision approaches need labor-intensive and time-consuming preprocessing and feature creation. The correctness of the learning method and features creation decides the success of

26

proposed method. The identification impact, however, was not as good as planned due to a lack of use of disease texture and color features.

Helly et al. (2003) [31] introduced a new technique in which the input picture is first converted to a Hue Saturation Intensity (HSI) color format, further, the Fuzzy C-mean technique was applied to separate the infected part from the image. The "shape, size, and color" characteristics of infected lesions were obtained and finally, these extracted features were fed into ANN for disease identification and classification. Authors claimed that the proposed system was 97 percent accurate.

In 2004, Moshou et al. (2004) [32] used Multilayer perceptron and Self-organisation map to detect yellow rust disease in wheat. wheat infection is recognized by using reflectance measurements. At an initial phase of yellow rust infection, spectral reflectance of infected and healthy plants was examined. Next, the variation in spectral reflectance of infected and healthy plant was explored. between healthy and sick wheat plants was explored in this study. A spectrograph placed at spray boom level was used to capture in-field spectral pictures. The researchers devised a normalisation approach based on light intensity adjustments and reflectance. Based on SOM, a unique approach for explaining interrelationships between variables and visualising data characteristics is described. On the basis of neural networks, disease identification technique has been built. An accuracy of 99% was achieved in the result analysis.

Sammany and Medhat (2007) [33] introduced a plant disease detection system based on a roughset approach to minimize the dimensions of extracted color and morphological features. In this paper, An ANN-based classifier was utilized to detect plant illnesses. The plant symptoms were classified using a neural network based on the leaf spot classes. Discolored (D), red-spotted (RS), white-spotted (WS), and Yellow-spotted (YS) are the four main classes. A set of discriminating factors are retrieved from a segmented leaf picture and afterward utilized for classification in order to identify the leaf spot class. These discriminating factors correspond to the spots' color and morphological properties. First, they improved the parameters using roughset approach and the design of neural networks using genetic algorithms. Then optimized neural networks along with SVM were employed to recognize the diseases of the plants. As seen in the result analysis, all of the situations resulting from the rough sets technique had greater accuracy (90 percent) than utilizing the entire feature set. This suggests that decreasing the number of features enhanced MLP's generalization ability while having no effect on the classification accuracy.

Meunkaewjinda et al. (2008) [34] proposed a technique for diagnosing grape plant illnesses. This method is based on image classification and detection techniques. The suggested method was divided into three sections: In the first step, the color of the leaf was retrieved from the complicated surrounding of leaf picture, in second step, the infected region's color was extracted, In the last step, the disease was classified.

In this study, a BPNN was combined with a SOFM to distinguish grape leaf colors. MSOFM and GA were also used to segment the leaf infection. Finally, Gabor Wavelet was used to filter the segmented picture, and SVM is used to categorize the leaf infection of the grape plant. Three classes of grape leaf were used to conduct the experiment. These classes are; healthy, rust disease, and scab disease. Despite the fact that there are several limits to retrieving color pixels from the image's background. For any farm products evaluation, the technique has shown to be quite promising.

In 2009, Li et al. (2009) [35] used Probabilistic Neural Network (PNN) to identify 2 types of diseases namely rice leaf roller and Aphelenchoides besseyi Christie found in rice plants. PNNs are a type of feedforward neural network that uses Parzen windows as its foundation. The activities of a PNN are grouped into a 4-layer feedforward network. Two types of spectral bands (visible and Shortwave Infrared) information were processed using PNN to detect the diseases. PCA approach was applied to form principal component spectrum by using the visible and Shortwave Infrared bands. Result analysis illustrated that the proposed system had a 95.65% accuracy rate in predicting illness and insect infection. Large memory requirement is drawback of PNN model.

Liu et al. (2009) [36] suggested a technique for distinguishing the healthy and sick parts of rice leaves using a BPNN as a classifier. Brown spot disease was chosen to investigate the proposed technique in this study. The input values to the BP neural network were color properties of healthy and diseased regions. The findings suggest that this technique may be used to diagnose other illnesses as well.

Al-Hiary et al. (2011) [37] presented an ANN-based crop disease recognition and categorization approach. The underlying principle that serves as the foundation in every computer vision classification system is nearly identical. First, a digital camera was utilized to collect digital photos from the interested farms. The obtained pictures are then subjected to image processing techniques in order to identify valuable information for next study. The photos are then classified using a variety of classification approaches based on the particular application. Here, Tiny whiteness, Late scorch, Ashen mould, Cottony mould, and Early scorch are the five illnesses considered for the study. The RGB pictures of leaves were transformed into the CIE Lab format. To locate the sick section of the leaf, the K-means approach was utilized. The Green section of the leaf was masked in the original picture. For feature extraction, the diseased areas are transformed to Hue saturation intensity format. The hue and saturation component of the HSI format was used to produce spatial grey level dependence matrices. "Texture features" were obtained and fed in the ANN classification model. Finally, classification task is completed using a NN. Authors claimed that suggested technique was 94% accurate. Similar approach was applied by Mrunalini et al. to recognise plant diseases.

Mrunalini et al. (2011) [38] proposed an ANN-based "disease detection and classification technique" to identify the diseases affecting the plant leaves. This types of automatic detection of diseases are very useful for farmers as it saves time, money, effort, and the environment. They have applied 3 image pre-processing operations (cropping, smoothing, and image enhancement) to enhance the visual appearance of input leaves images. Thresholding and binarization are used to segment and locate leaf parts from the back-ground. Diseased regions were obtained by masking the green pixels. In masking operation, first of all, green pixels were identified. Then a threshold value (which corresponds to minimum intraclass variance) was computed by applying the global thresholding method. The intensity of the pixel was cleared if the green part of the pixel is less than the calculated threshold. Further, the pixels with zero intensity are eliminated. The feature extraction procedure was applied to infected regions. Authors have used the "color co-occurrence method (CCM)" to extract the necessary attributes from leaves to classify the diseases. Texture and color features were used in the features extraction process. These "extracted features" were fed into ANN to automatically detect and classify the diseases. They have claimed that their suggested method performed well.

In 2011, Image processing methods are used by Kai et al. (2011) [39] to study illnesses diagnosis and classification for maize plants. They have acquired leaves images of maze plants to conduct the experiments. To locate the infected lesions, "RGB" images of maze leaf were transformed into "YCbCr color format". YCbCr color space approach was used to segment infected spots from leaf images. Further, the "Co-occurrence matrix" method was applied on the infected spot to get texture features of diseased regions. A backpropagation neural network architecture was applied on extracted features to identify maze diseases. VC++ platform was utilized to conduct the experiments. Result analysis indicated that the proposed system effectively recognizes the leaf diseases. Suggested model was found 98 percent accurate.

Further, Kulkarni et al. (2012) [40] introduced a "plant disease detection" technique by applying image processing on plant leaf images. Diseased leaves of pomegranate plants were acquired for the study. They have included 3 diseases (Bacterial blight, alterneria, and Anthractnose) in this research. 89 instances of Anthractnose , 26 instances of Bacterial blight, and 8 instances of alterneria were used as input dataset to conduct the experiments. Gabor filter was utilized to discover relevant classification features from leaf images. These extracted attributes were used by ANN classifier for automatic disease classification. ANN with 50 hidden neurons has given optimum results. Authors have implemented the experiments at different termination error and found that termination error of 0.00001 gave best recognition rate. Total 4500 iterations were applied during training and testing of the classifier. Gradient was set on 0.02. During validation of ANN at optimum setup, recognition rate of alterneria was recorded as 81.5%, whereas recognition rates of Bacterial blight and Anthractnose were recorded as 94% and 97.5% respectively. Thus, an overall recognition rate of 91% was achieved in the result analysis.

Wang et al. (2012) [41] demonstrated plant disease recognition system using the dataset from 2 crops, wheat, and grape. A total of 185 digital photos were evaluated, with 85 leaf samples of grape and 100 leaf samples of wheat. The photos are downsized using the NearestNeighbour interpolation approach without affecting the image resolution.

To remove noises from the photos, the median-filter was used. For segmentation, the K-means algorithm was utilized. The RGB picture was transformed to CIE XYZ color format before performing the segmentation. Further, the XYZ color format was transformed to Lab format. Features such as "texture, shape, and color" were retrieved. The dimensionality of the feature was minimized by using principal component analysis (PCA). Reduced features set requires a smaller number of neurons in the NN and hence speed up the training and validation of the suggested model. BPNN was used as a classifier to classify the diseases.

Jaware et al. (2012) [42] proposed an accurate and fast approach for plant disease detection and categorization. Cottony mould, early scorch, ashen mould, small whitening, and late scorch are the 5 principal plant diseases that the suggested strategy is evaluated on. The RGB picture was first captured after which the acquired RGB image was transformed by establishing a transformation structure. Following that, RGB color values were changed to the space defined in the color transformation structure.

The segmentation process is then carried out utilizing the Kmeans clustering approach. The primarily green pixels are then covered. Furthermore, the diseased

31

cluster was identified by eliminating the green color. The infected cluster was then transformed from RGB to HSI color structure. The SGDM matrices were then constructed for each pixel map of the picture for just HSI images in the next stage. At the final stage, a pre-trained ANN was used to recognize the retrieved feature. The findings demonstrate that the suggested system can accurately identify and categorize illnesses with an accuracy of 83 percent to 94 percent.

Owomugisha et al. (2014) [43] introduced an automatic diseases detection method for the banana plants. They have worked on Black Sigatoka and Bacterial Wilt Diseases in their study. Authors claimed that ML has been used in farming in a variety of fields, notably plant disease diagnosis and the development of image processing systems for particular crops. The examples of such crops are Cassava, potatoes, tomatoes, wheat, sugar cane, vegetables, grapes, pomegranate and Cotton. Further they added that no ML approaches were used to try to identify infections in banana crop such as banana black sigatoka (BBS) and banana bacterial wilt (BBW), due to which farmers lost a lot of money. This research examined varieties of computer vision approaches, and developed a system consisting of 4 major parts to identify banana diseases. In first part, Photos of banana leaves were taken using digital camera. In second part, multiple feature extraction approaches were utilised to acquire important data that will be utilized in part three. Part three was implemented to perform the classification. Performance assessment was done in last fourth part.

Authors have retrieved color histograms and converted them from RGB to HSV and from RGB to L*a*b format. Max tree was created using peak components. The area under the curve and five attributes related to shape were used to classify the diseases.

Input image samples have experimented with several classifiers namely support vector machine, Naïve Bayes, extremely randomized Tree, random forest, Decision tree, and nearest neighbours. Extremely randomized trees offer high accuracy among others. Extremely Randomized Trees have given best result with an area under the curve (AUC) of 0.91 for BBS and 0.96 for BBW among the 7 experimented classifiers. To judge the effectiveness of experimented classification models AUC was used.

Khirade and Patil (2015) [44] presented a study that looked at several machine learning and image processing strategies for detecting plant illnesses through leaf photos. The authors have presented 5 steps solution for plant disease detection and classification. They have not illustrated any experiment in their study but only discussed the possible methods used for the detection of plant leaf diseases. First of all, they suggested a color conversion structure, then discussed a colour space conversion that was device-independent. In the second step, Contrast enhancement, picture smoothing, histogram equalization, and clipping pre-processing techniques were discussed to get better visual characteristics for input images. Further, In the third step, they have discussed K-means segmentation, lesion recognition, boundary identification, and Otsu's thresholding segmentation techniques in their study. These segmentation techniques were presented to get infected regions in the input images. In the fourth step, they have presented various features extraction techniques in their study. Color, edges, morphology, and texture are among the key discriminating parameters that were highlighted in the paper. The color co-occurrence Method was discussed for achieving unique features related to color and texture from the images. SGDM was suggested to perform the statistical calculations on texture to extract texture features by applying Gray Level Co-occurrence Matrix (GLCM). In the final step, the disease detection and classification approach with ANN was described.

In 2015, Rastogi et al. (2015) [45] presented fuzzy logic and computer vision-based disease recognition and grading techniques. Using DIP and ML techniques, this research presents a simple and efficient technique for identifying and categorizing leaf illness. The suggested method consisted of 2 phases. The first phase involves pre-processing of leaves pictures and extraction of features, succeeded by ANN classification model to recognize the leaf. The illness existing in the leaves was classified in the 2nd phase, which involves the "K-Means" technique to segment the infected regions followed by features extraction and then disease classification.

GLCM was utilized to retrieve texture information. Disease classification was done using ANN. The illness is then graded based on the intensity of disease found in the sample. Fuzzy logic was applied to grade the illness.

In 2015, Sannakki and Rajpurohit (2015) [46] suggested a disease classification model for the Pomegranate plant. They devised a strategy that was mainly based on the segmentation scheme. Pomegranate leaves were used to provide learning to the developed model. A digital camera was used to capture pictures of normal and diseased leaves samples. To find contaminated parts, the visual appearance of image was improved and segmented. The proposed method applied segmentation technique to locate the defective region and then discovered the texture and color properties of infected lesions. These extracted properties were used as classification features. The categorization was done with the help of an ANN classifier. The classification accuracy was determined to be 97.30%. The biggest drawback is that it can only be utilized for a small number of harvests.

Rothe and Kshirsagar (2015) [47] presented a pattern recognition approach for the diagnosis of infections found in the leaves of the cotton plants. Cotton plant leaf diseases must be recognised early and correctly, since they might have a negative impact on the production. Alternaria, Myrothecium, and Bacterial Blight diseases have been recognized and categorized using a PR system in the suggested study. Images for this study were taken directly from the crop fields located at 3 different regions. First site was chosen as crop field of cotton plant located at Nagpur (Central Institute of Cotton Research). Second and third sites were chosen as crop fields of Wardha and Buldana districts, respectively. They have used snake segmentation to separate infected sections and then used Hu's moments as a distinguishing feature. The "active contour model" was utilized to restrict the vitality within the diseased lesion, and the Backpropagation neural network architecture was used to solve a variety of classification issues. The average accuracy of 85.52 percent was achieved by the suggested model.

Further, Ghaiwat et al. (2014) [48] have presented a study of the many classification approaches that may be utilized to classify plant leaf diseases. This work gives an idea of the advantages and disadvantages of several strategies that may be utilized to recognize and classify leaf diseases. A classification strategy involves categorizing each pattern into one of distinct categories. Classification is a method of classifying leaves based on their shape, color, and texture characteristics. ANN and Fuzzy logic, PCA, SVM, Genetic Algorithm (GA), Probabilistic Neural Network (PNN), and k-Nearest Neighbour classifiers were a few well-known examples among available classification algorithms which were discussed in the study. They have realized that choosing a classification technique was really challenging work since the effectiveness of the performance varied depending on the nature of the input samples. For the provided validation cases, the k-NN approach appeared to be the most appropriate and straightforward in all given methods. Further, the author has added limitations of SVM. They have observed that it was challenging to find appropriate parameters in SVM if the data used for model training was not linearly separable, that seems to be its shortcoming.

In 2015, Mokhtar et al. (2015) [49] applied SVM to recognize 2 types of viruses found in tomato leaves. They employed an SVM classifier with varying kernels to the segmented sick parts and used several color and shape-based characteristics. "Tomato yellow leaf curl virus (TYLCV)" is among the most dangerous viruses, causing TYLCV disease around the globe. It leads to yellowing and upward curling of tomato leaves. This study outlines a method for detecting and identifying diseased leaves infected with 2 viruses named "Tomato spotted wilt virus (TSWV) and Tomato yellow leaf curl virus (TYLCV)". "Pre-processing, picture segmentation, feature extraction, and classification are the four primary aspects of the suggested technique". Segmentation was applied to each leaf picture, and a description for every segment is generated. To choose the best features, several geometric metrics were used. For disease categorization, an SVM method with various kernel functions was utilized. 200 contaminated leaves pictures with TYLCV and TSWV were utilized to train and validate the proposed model. The results of the provided strategy are evaluated using the N-fold cross-validation technique. According to the findings of the experiments, the suggested classification strategy had an average accuracy of 90% and a quadratic kernel function accuracy of 92 percent.

Further, Vishnu et al. (2015) [50] examined and discussed the image processing strategies for identifying diseases in plants. They have reviewed various "pre-processing, image segmentation, and feature extraction techniques". Segmentation based on different aspects was discussed in this research paper. They have talked about "model-based segmentation like Markov Random Field (MRF) based segmentation, threshold-based segmentation, edge-based segmentation, region-based segmentation, and clustering-based segmentation". For features extraction, authors have discussed PCA, Gabor filters, Wavelet transform, GLCM, and SGDM techniques. The authors said that BPNN, SGDM, Kmeans algorithm, and SVM are the most familiar methods for detecting the infection in plant leaves. These methods can be utilized to examine the leaves of both normal and sick plants. Further, they discussed the 3 challenges coming during the implementation of these techniques. These challenges are automation of the suggested approach for uninterrupted persistent surveillance of crop diseases under actual field settings, optimization of the approach for particular plant diseases, and the influence of background information in the generated picture samples. According to the review, "these approaches have a lot of potential including the capacity to identify leaf illnesses and certain drawbacks". As a result, there is room for enhancement in the present approaches.

After presenting the review, the authors have proposed a disease recognition and classification method. First, they converted RGB images into HSV image format. Then K-means algorithm was utilized to segment leaves before calculating texture characteristics for the separated diseased items. Finally, a neural network classifier was used to process the extracted features.

Using photos of damaged and normal leaves, Prajapati et al. (2017) [51] developed an SVM-based diagnosis system to diagnose illnesses in rice plants. They employed

36

DIP algorithms on input samples to obtain a high-quality picture and then used ML to create a disease prediction model based on pre-processed samples. The background of the sample pictures was removed during pre-processing. To find the sick region of the leaves, they employed the Kmeans clustering technique. "The size, color, and texture information" of damaged parts of the leaf were utilized as indicators of illness. The suggested approach has a training sample accuracy of 93.33 percent and a test sample accuracy of 73.33 percent.

Using rice leaf digital photographs, Jayanti et al. (2019) [52] built a prediction system to diagnose rice leaves illness. DIP techniques were used to remove noises from the image samples and to locate the infected regions in leaf images. To remove noises from the input image samples, a median filter has been used. These pre-processing operations helped to achieve high-quality photographs of rice leaves. The fuzzy C-mean clustering approach was used to find the borders of sick sections. Speeded-up robust features (SURF) and texturing approaches were used to retrieve important features from infected regions of input samples.

To diagnose illnesses, these collected features were fed into an ANN model to recognize and categorize the diseases. They claimed to obtain a good outcome but did not specify the method's exact accuracy.

Crop disease identification algorithms depend on capturing several types of information from infected plant leaves photos. Leaf infections are key factors because it significantly reduces the amount and quality of farming products. As a result, diagnosing and comprehending illnesses are essential. In conclusion we can say that presented reviews generally suggest two steps to recognising diseases based on leaf images: First collecting morphological, texture, and color attributes from infected regions (ii) applying ML algorithms to categorise unhealthy leaf samples. Similar approach was also utilised by Nandhini et al. (2020) [53]. Based on the collected attributes, this study examined the efficiency of categorization of diseases using decision Trees, SVM, and KNN.

2.1.3 Related to DL Approaches for "Plant Disease Recognition and Classification" without Transfer Learning

DNN have been shown to improve the result in a variety of image processing, Natural language processing, classification, and image recognition tasks, therefore many researchers decided to use them for object detection. For classification by extracting relevant features, researchers employed a DNN variation called Deep CNN. The beauty of Deep CNN is its ability to learn the relevant features automatically. It can be utilized for both classification and features extraction. Many authors used deep CNN for both purposes features capturing and classification [santosh upadhyay]. While many other researchers used Deep CNN only for features extraction and then they performed classification using several ML techniques (ANN, SVM, KNN, decision tree, etc.) [54]. The application of deep CNN does not remain unnoticed in the field of agriculture. Agriculture scientists and researchers have started to use Deep Learning (CNN) techniques to solve various agricultural problems like crop yield detection, weed detection, crop monitoring, leaf detection, and crop disease detection. In these problems, crop disease is a major problem since crop yields are greatly impacted by plant diseases. In this subsection, I have outlined various deep learning techniques used in crop illness recognition and categorization.

Deep learning is increasingly gaining attraction as the efficient and effective method for picture categorization. The biggest challenge in applying this method to automatically identify crop diseases is a shortage of picture datasets that can reflect the large range of symptom and conditions of features encountered in reality. Data augmentation approaches reduce the effect of this issue. But many times, data augmentations are unable to recreate the majority of the practical variation. Rather than evaluating the full leaf, some research investigates the application of particular patches and lesions for the purpose. The variety of the input sample is raised with no requirement of additional photographs because each affected area has its unique features. It also makes it possible to identify several illnesses that affect the same leaf. Barbedo (2013) [55] has used this type of approach to automatically diagnose the plant diseases.

Lue et al. (2018) [56] proposed a deep learning technique to recognize apple diseases found in China. Based on deep convolutional neural networks, this research provided an accurate identification strategy for apple leaves infection. To identify apple leaf illnesses, it deals with obtaining the diseased pictures and constructing a unique structure of a Deep CNN based on the architecture of AlexNet. They have designed suggested architecture by merging alexnet with inception modules.

Nesterov's Accelerated Gradient optimization was preferred in the training process in place of Stochastic Gradient Descent (SGD) optimization, due to to its nature of higher rate of convergence. To illustrate the effectiveness of Nesterov's Accelerated Gradient, they have evaluated their model with SGD and Nesterov's Accelerated Gradient optimizers and found that the SGD optimizer gave an accuracy of 93.32% while Nesterov's Accelerated Gradient had given 97.62 percent accuracy.

The suggested model was trained to recognize the 4 prevalent apple leaves illnesses using a collection of 13,689 photos of sick leaves. The validation results demonstrated that the suggested CNN-based model attained 97.62 percent overall validation accuracy. They have found that the parameters of the model were lowered by 51,206,928 when matched with basic Alexnet architecture while classification accuracy improved by 10.83 percent.

This study found that the suggested CNN model offers a superior infection prevention strategy for illnesses found in the apple plant. They also observed that higher accuracy was achieved at a faster rate due to the use of Nesterov's Accelerated Gradient optimizer.

Agarwal et al. (2020) [57] suggested a simple deep CNN structure namely ToLeD to recognize tomato leaf illnesses. They have evaluated the performance of the suggested model on the leaf samples of tomato from the PlantVillage dataset. The performance analysis of ToLeD was done in comparison with other well-known deep CNN architectures namely InceptionV3, VGG16, and MobileNet and it was noticed that the developed system behaved well and showed better accuracy than that of the other model. Classification accuracy of 91.2% was obtained.

The major issue in using the deep learning (DL) method to automatically recognize crop diseases is a shortage of picture datasets that can reflect the large range of symptoms and conditions of features encountered in reality. In this research, a modified extended dataset was proposed by Barbedo (2019) [58] to reduce this issue which consists of a sample of individual spots and lesions rather than leaf images. They have included 79 diseases related to 14 plant varieties in their research to create this data set. Here segmentation process was still performed manually to locate infected parts, which prevent the complete automation. The accuracy acquired with this method was on average 12% greater than the accuracy obtained using the actual photos. Furthermore, disease classification accuracy did not drop less than 75 percent for any crop, even though 10 illnesses were taken into account. The author said that even though the suggested dataset did not capture the complete range of real situations, still, findings of result analysis showed that deep learning approaches are accurate for detecting and recognizing plant diseases as long as adequate data is provided.

Further, Trivedi et al. (2021) [59] proposed CNN based disease diagnosis system for tomato crops. We know that tomatoes are among the most important and widely consumed vegetables on the planet. The quantity of tomatoes varies depending on how they are cultivated. Leaf infections are the most significant factor affecting crop production quantity and quality. Therefore, it's crucial to accurately identify and categorize these illnesses. Tomato yields are badly impacted by a variety of illnesses. Early detection of such deadly diseases would help to lessen the infection's impact on crops and increase crop production. Various novel methods of categorizing specific diseases had been extensively used.

The goal of this study [59] was to assist farm owners in reliably diagnosing initial crops infections and alerting the farmers. To properly recognize and categorize infections found in tomato leaves, the Convolutional Neural Network (CNN) was used. CNN-based segmentation technique was applied to RGB images to get masked images. This masked image was divided into small square regions. Then the area of interest was chosen from these square regions. These areas of interest were utilized to obtain features related to texture, shape, and color automatically using CNN classifier. The entire investigation was done using Google Collaborative and a database including 3000 photos of tomato leaves infected with 9 different illnesses as well as a normal leaf. The following is a detailed description of the entire procedure: The input photographs are first segmented using CNN, and the infected regions of the images were captured. Next, the photographs are also treated using different CNN hyper-parameters. Finally, deep CNN pulls various features from images, including edges, texture, and color. The outcomes illustrated that the suggested model's diagnosis was 98.49% correct.

The training of a deep convolutional neural network (DCNN) needs a large amount of data; however, data availability is an issue in agriculture. Many times, researchers used the augmentation technique to increase the size of the dataset and to achieve variations in input samples. To enhance the precision of plant disease diagnosis, a lightweight disease detection model for tomato plants backed by Variational Auto-Encoder (VAE) was suggested by Wu et al. (2021) [60]. Multi-scale convolution in the lightweight network can widen the network, and enrich the retrieved features. The parameters like deep separable convolution were reduced by this proposed network. VAE achieves unsupervised learning by utilizing a huge amount of unlabelled data and afterward employs labeled data for supervised illness detection.

The recognition accuracy and generalization impact of the suggested model was improved when compared to a model that only employs labeled data. The detection performance has grown from 56.13 percent to 78.03 percent, even with smaller labeled data, and it has also increased in the case of more labeled instances. The performance of the lightweight proposed model backed with the VAE improvement approach has been fully confirmed. The suggested technique has a 94.17 percent classification accuracy with only 0.42 percent of infected leaves misclassified as normal leaves. The classification accuracy of healthy samples was 98.27 percent, with only 1.73 percent of normal samples misclassified as infected leaves.

Verma and Dubey (2021) [61] proposed a unique video processing-based technique for illness identification in rice leaf. Suggested method included 2 deep learning architectures: LSTM and RNN. A cell phone was used to record videos of rice plants. The recorded movies were split into 2 sections one was utilised for validation and other for testing. The collected films were segmented using colour indexing with linear colour space transformation. Time-series datasets consisting of fuzzy, entropy and standard deviation attributes were retrieved after video image segmentation.

The suggested LSTM-RNN-based system for detecting sick and healthy rice plants was trained using derived dataset. The developed model was stated to have a prediction accuracy of 99.99 percent by the author. In addition, the proposed technique.

Kumbhar et al. (2019) [62] created a system for disease classification in cotton crops using Deep CNN. A cotton leaf picture collection was used to provide training to the classifier. 720 leaf photos of the cotton plant were obtained, including 513 instances to train and 207 instances to test the classifier. The obtained photos were resized to make them 128 *128 pixels wide. CNN was built to capture the discriminating attributes from the input leaf photo automatically. To capture the discriminating attributes from pictures CL was used as first hidden layer. To reduce the size of feature map, the PL was applied at next layer. Completely linked layer was used at third position to flatten the network. The suggested framework was 80 percent accurate during training whereas 89% accurate during validation.

Bodapati et al. (2019) [54] used Deep CNN only for features extraction and then they performed classification using the SVM technique. They have conducted 2 experiments. In the first experiment, they have developed a deep CNN model with 3 hidden layers for features extraction. Then captured attributes were given as input to NN with 2 hidden layers to perform the classification. In the second experiment, they have performed feature capturing and categorization using 2 different models. In the second experiment, first, significant features were captured using the Deep CNN model then extracted features were fed into the SVM classifier to complete the classification task. The results of both experiments were evaluated. The results of SVM based categorization on CNN based extracted features in experiment 2 were marginally better than the performance of NN based classification achieved in experiment 1.

In both theoretical and practical aspects, CNNs are a useful pattern identification approach. Using deep learning, Lu et al. (2017) [63] offer a novel method for improving CNNs' learning potential. Through image identification, the presented CNNs-based Network can accurately categorize ten prevalent paddy illnesses. The implementation of the suggested CNNs model in the diagnosis of paddy diseases demonstrates that it can effectively and accurately identify plant infection. The suggested technique outperforms the other model in terms of identification ability, convergence rate, and training accuracy. They have used ten deadly diseases found in paddy crops. 500 pictures of healthy and unhealthy leaves were gathered directly from the rice crop field. A 10-fold cross-validation technique was used to deal with the problem of overfitting. 95.48 percent accuracy was recorded in the result analysis.

The authors have applied stochastic pooling operation in place of mean/max pooling in CNN architecture. To demonstrate the effectiveness of stochastic pooling, the authors experimented with the same model on the same dataset with mean polling and max-pooling one by one. Result analysis indicated that the stochastic pooling operation gave a better result than the other 2 arrangements. The authors have also analyzed the performance of the suggested model with different filter sizes and outlined their accuracies in the research paper.

43

Using photos of contaminated rice plants, the Patidar et al. (2020) [64] proposed a method for detecting and classifying infections in rice crop, that is most important and preferable grains in the India. Three types of diseases were studied in this research. Dataset were acquired from the UCI Machine Learning Repository. Residual Neural Network (RNN) was utilized to perform recognition and categorization of diseases. They have compared performance of suggested RNN based model with Simple CNN and SVM and found that proposed system outperforms than other 2 compared methods. They claimed that RNN prevent to touch saturation mark, even with large datasets.

.2.1.4 Related to Deep Learning Approaches for Plant Disease Recognition and Classification with Transfer Learning

Agriculture is a common domain that is susceptible to viral, bacterial and fungus illness.

To increase agricultural productivity, crop diseases must be detected accurately and early. The Deep learning is useful in detecting crop diseases utilising a large quantity of plant leaf photos. Convolution Neural Network (CNN) is among the most widely used architectures in deep learning. But, utilising deep learning approaches to recognise illness with limited and small databases is a difficult task. One of the most prominent deep learning algorithms for correctly detecting the plant illnesses with small dataset is transfer learning. Deep convolution neural network model based on transfer learning is proposed by the researchers for disease identification in various crops.

In this subsection, we have presented literature review of various research papers that focus their study on transfer learning.

Zhang et al. (2018) [65] used deep learning techniques to provide maize disease detection system. They felt that the automated detection and characterization of diseases found in maize leaves are widely wanted in the domain of agriculture. Therefore, the revised Cifar10 and GoogLeNet deep learning architectures were suggested for maize leaf disease recognition in this study to increase detection performance and minimize the number of model parameters. Modifying the pooling choices, incorporating ReLu layers and dropout processes, tuning the network parameters, and lowering the number of classifiers result in two better models that were utilized to train and evaluate 9 different types of maize leaf pictures. Furthermore, the enhanced architectures have a substantially lower number of parameters than the AlexNet and VGG architectures. The GoogLeNet architecture has an average accuracy rate of 98.9% when recognizing 8 types of diseases in maize plants, whereas the Cifar10 architecture obtained 98.8% average accuracy.

Transfer learning strategy is not only being used in leaf disease recognition, but also being used by different researchers in recognition of plant types.

One such experiment was conducted by Ghazi et al. (2017) [66] to detect the species of plants.In their work, Ghazi et al. employ deep CNN models to recognize the plants types for given leaf picture. They have investigated different network parameters and assessed the effects of various parameters on the results of these models. This task of plant recognition was accomplished using 3 successful and well-known CNN variants: VGGNet, AlexNet,, and GoogLeNet. LifeCLEF 2015 plant task databases were utilised to apply transfer learning on these pre-trained networks. Problem of overfitting was minimised by applying data augmentation. To boost overall accuracy, the hyperparameters of networks were modified and CNNs are fused. Suggested system achieved validation accuracy of 80%.

InceptionResNetV2 is a form of CNN architecture that was used with a transfer learning strategy to recognize leaf diseases by Krishnamoorthy et al. (2021) [67]. The parameters of suggested model were tuned in such a good manner that they achieved a high accuracy of 95.67 percent. This study takes into account 4 classes of leaf samples: healthy class as well as 3 diseased classes (bacterial blight, leaf blast, brown spot). The authors have implemented 2 experiments to show the effectiveness of transfer learning. One experiment was conducted with simple CNN and the other with InceptionResNetV2. By performing fifteen epochs, multiple network parameters were tested on basic CNN and reached an accuracy of 84.75 percent. On the other hand, by applying ten epochs with transfer learning InceptionResNetV2 was able to achieve an optimal accuracy of 95.67 percent.

Chen et al. (2020) [68] investigated Deep CNN architectures with a transfer learning approach for the detection of leaf diseases. Already trained CNN models were used to initialize the weight and biases of a suggested network. In this study, VGGNet pre-trained model was used with the inception module. These pre-trained networks were trained on huge data set namely ImageNet. On the public repository, the suggested technique obtains a test accuracy of at least 91.83 percent, which is a significant enhancement over previous state-of-the-art approaches. The suggested technique achieves an average classification accuracy of 92.00 percent even with a noisy background. Experiments show that the suggested technique is viable and that it may be used to identify plant diseases quickly.

Tomato is a common food item that is susceptible to illness. The introduction of ML and deep learning (DL) approaches have made it simpler to identify agricultural diseases. Sangeetha et al. (2020) [69] introduced a transfer learning strategy using 2 deep learning architecture namely VGG19 and VGG16. DL has become a strong technology for data analytics and image processing in recent times, with promising outcomes. DL has been used in a wide range of fields, notably farming. Convolution Neural Network (CNN) is among the most widely used architectures in deep learning. Transfer learning is a novel method in deep learning that uses pre-trained architecture to train a fresh database to speed up the learning process. The goal of this study is to create a Transfer Learning-driven classification model for detecting leaf illness. A novel composite and detailed prediction system for tomato disease assessment is established in this research. Proposed classification system was created by combining 2 DL models, namely VGG19 and VGG16. Accuracy, F1-score, recall, and Precision, were used to analyse the performance. The higher accuracy of Transfer Learning demonstrated in this published study supports its use in the disease classification and recognition.

In order to assist the farmers and crop owners for increasing the agricultural productivity, Thangaraj et al. (2021) [70] introduced a DCNN model based on TL for disease identification in tomato crops. The system detects disease by combining stored photos and real-time acquired pictures of the leaves of tomato plants. They have used 3 different kinds of optimizers one by one to check the performance of the proposed model. "RMSprop optimizers, stochastic gradient descent (SGD), and Adaptive moment estimation (Adam)", are used to assess the results of the suggested model. This exercise was done to get the best possible results and to analyse the effect of several optimizers on the suggested network. The validation results show that the suggested system, which employs a transfer learning technique, is accurate in classifying tomato diseases automatically. When contrasted to RMSprop and SGD optimizers, the Adam provides higher accuracy.

Further, Hasan et al. (2019) [71] felt that the farming industry in India is affected by challenges such as poor crop productivity, widespread usage of pesticides and fertilisers, outdated production practises. Using a CNN, Hasan et al. created a precision farming system based on drone to successfully detect high infectious region in a crop field. With the use of drones, they have planned to apply targeted insecticides on the infected region. Authors have collected 2100 samples from online sources and combined it with 500 samples captured from the crop fields. To develop the detection system, Google's inception model was retrained using transfer learning strategy. To decide the proper insecticide dosage, leaves are divided into three classes: bad, nominal, good. When the proportion of training dataset is raised to 85 percent, 99 percent accuracy is obtained.

Similar kind of approach was utilized by Abas et al. (2018) [72] to classify plant varieties. The possibility of using VGG16 deep architecture for plant categorization is discussed in this research. Due to similar characteristics of colour and shape of leaf of many plants, flower photos were utilised as input sample in place of leaves. Earlier studies have shown that employing data augmentation, dropout and transfer learning minimise the overfitting issue of deep network when used to a small set of samples. With 2800 flower photos, authors were able to effectively develop and train the VGG16 model. The model had a validation accuracy of 93.93%.

In Thailand, Mathulaprangsan et al. (2020) [73] attempted to solve the challenge of manual rice disease recognition. Authors suggested a two-phase rice disease identification paradigm. They began the research by capturing photos of rice plants in order to create the dataset. Then DenseNets and ResNets pre-trained deep learning (DL) architectures were used to categorize the rice illnesses in the second phase. On the collected datasets, some alternative DL architectures were also tested to compare the outcomes of the suggested strategy. The suggested model attained an average accuracy of 95% in experiments, according to the results. The authors say that their technique will be simple to adopt in the future and will be capable of helping Thai farmers.

To diagnose 4 kinds of rice diseases, Islam et al. (2021) [74] introduced a CNN-based automated disease recognition technique. Leaf smut, leaf blight, leaf blast and brown spot diseases were included in this study. To provide the learning to the CNN models, they have utilized healthy leaf photos as well as these unhealthy leaf images. The authors tested 4 types of CNN models: ResNet-101, Xception, VGG-19, and Inception-Resnet-V2. They discovered that Inception-ResNet-V2 outperformed the others. Inception-ResNet-V2 obtained an accuracy of 92.68 percent.

Jadhav et al. (2020) [75] introduced a pathogen recognition method for the soybean plants using a TL methodology. To create illness detection models, they utilised 2 deep CNN architectures (AlexNet and GoogleNet). They have created 2 detection models. The GoogleNet architecture was used in one model, while the AlexNet architecture was used in the other. The suggested system was developed using photos of soybean leaves that were obtained from dataset. The training set included 649 photos of sick leaves and 550 images of healthy leaves. The suggested system was put to the test on 80 very new leaf photos. In result analysis, GoogleNet-based model has given 96.25 percent accuracy while accuracy of AlexNet-based model was observed as 98.75%.

Further, Ghosal et al. (2020) [76] used a TL approach to develop a deep CNN model for rice illness identification. authors They have produced a little dataset of their own. The introduced CNN model was built utilising a VGG-16 architecture pre-trained-on massive dataset. Learned information was transferred to train and verify the proposed model using a field dataset that was created by the authors. Their recommended model has a 92.46 percent accuracy rate.

Deng et al. (2021) [77] suggested an ensemble learning strategy based on DL architectures for automated identification of 6 kinds of rice illnesses. Authors have conducted experiments with ensemble learning using several deep learning models. To verify the model, a large database of 33,026 photos was utilized. False smut, leaf blast, neck blast, bacterial stripe disease, sheath blight, and brown spot diseases were tested in this study. Ensemble learning using the ResNeSt50, DenseNet-121, and SE-ResNet-50 deep CNN models outperformed other methods in result analysis. The proposed strategy has a 91 percent accuracy.

2.2 Research Gap Identification

Various relevant studies related to plant disease diagnosis and classification are selected for literature review of this research. These studies have been published in various reputed journals and conferences. The main purpose of literature review is to recognize unexplored areas that could be further explored. The conclusion and future scope section of all reviewed research papers are carefully studied to identify the research gaps. We have identified following research gaps during the literature review:

1. In all the reviewed methods, very few methods have given 99% or more accuracy.

2. Since maximum of the benchmarked plant disease dataset consists of image samples labelled with disease name only, but not contains image samples labelled with disease intensity or severity. To overcome this issue, an infection severity estimation method can be developed to derive new dataset labelled with disease intensity from existing plant disease dataset.

3. Even with small datasets and complex background images, better accuracy can be achieved.

2.3 Research Objectives

1. Review of the literatures to find the limitations of the most effective methods utilized in plant leaf disease detection and severity estimation.

2. Propose a novel deep learning approach to detect deadly rice diseases with aim of enhancing detection accuracy and reducing the error rate by using proposed deep CNN architecture.

3. Develop an infection severity estimation method based on two phase image segmentation technique to derive new dataset labelled with disease intensity from existing plant disease dataset.

4. Propose an effective brown spot disease recognition and classification model capable of capturing the infection at early stage.

5. Develop the transfer learning models to enhance the disease detection and classification accuracy even with small dataset and complex background images.

CHAPTER 3

RICE PLANT LEAF DISEASE DIAGNOSIS MODEL USING IMAGE PROCESSING AND DEEP CNN ARCHITECTURE

3.1 Introduction

Agricultural production occupies a very important place in a developing country like India. The livelihood of many people of the country depends on agriculture related occupation. Near about 70 percent of India's people maintain their livelihood from agriculture [78]. Rice is one of the important grains among agricultural crops. Rice is eaten in many countries of the world. Most of the people in India like rice as their favorite food [79]. Rice and its related food products contribute a lot to India's economy. In India, paddy is cultivated over a large area from east to west and north to south. There are many factors that can reduce the yield of rice, in which the soil factor, biological factor, environmental factor, and seed selection are important factors. If any one of these factors is not balanced then it leads to plant disease. Rice diseases are very dangerous and harmful, it reduces the production by about ten to fifteen percent every year in India [80]. The main sources of plant diseases are viral infections, bacterial infections and fungal infections. This disease can affect any part of the plant. These parts include the plant's root, stem, leaves, flowers and fruits. If these diseases are not recognized and treated in time, then they ruin the entire crop. Traditionally these diseases are identified by seeing them through the eyes and analysing them manually. This manual method is bias and sometimes it is inaccurate. Farmers sometimes do not recognize rice disease correctly and sometimes they misidentify, that leads greater loss to the crop yields. In recent times, there has been a lot of improvement in machine learning, deep learning and image processing techniques Researchers and agricultural scientists are using these technologies for plant disease diagnosis and categorization now a days. BLB, Leaf smut and BS are the most frequent infections affecting rice plant [81], Al-Bashish (2011) [82].

Many plants disease diagnosis system based on digital image processing as discussed by Barbedo (2013) [55], computer vision as discussed by Khairnar (2014) [83], and pattern recognition as discussed by Phadikar (2008) [84], have been developed by various researchers to achieve efficient and effective disease prediction system. A smart equipment can be deployed in the agriculture field to gain benefits of such detection systems. Camera sensors can be installed at different spots throughout the farm field to gather plant images. These sensors take photographs at periodic times, and the detection system analyses the images to see if the plant is infected. Farmers benefit greatly from such systems because they receive timely and correct knowledge on plant diseases.

In general, machine learning Shruthi (2019) [85] / variants of ML (DL) and DIP are the 2 main building elements of any plant disease diagnosis system. Leaf samples from plants are either gathered from a well-known source repository that has been tested or taken from agricultural fields. We have used rice disease leaf samples in our studies.

DIP is a method of processing and displaying digital pictures using a computer and an appropriate algorithm. Image processing is used on pictures to conduct various operations (such as background and noise reduction, image segmentation, image scaling, image transformation, image resizing and feature extraction, etc.) in order to achieve a certain purpose. The goal of our research is to use image processing and deep learning to diagnose rice plant illnesses.

Machine learning method is used in computer vision to detect and classify important elements in photographs. Machine learning is utilized to create a classification or predictive model that is developed to learn using training data and then evaluated to predict or classify an unseen input. Deep learning is a new technique for extracting features from leaf photos automatically. Deep Convolution neural network (DCNN) has been a growing topic for picture categorization due to its ability to extract features automatically. It can manage applications related to big data without the need for picture pre-processing. A fundamental step required to build a plant disease identification and classification system using ML is depicted in Figure 3.1.

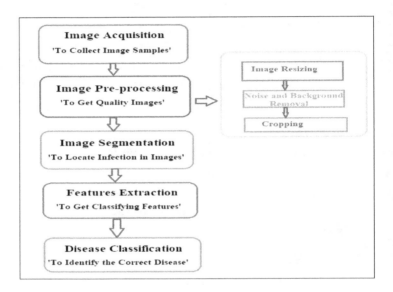

Figure 3.1 Flow diagram for plant leaf disease detection using ML

1. Image Acquisition: The initial stage in every image processing programme is image acquisition. The goal of image capture is to gather pictures of the plant's sick parts. The photos are obtained either from a benchmarked dataset or from the crop field in this stage. The photographs collected are used as train and test samples.

2. Image Pre-processing: The dataset is cleaned using image pre-processing techniques. Image pre-processing entails a variety of procedures that are carried out according to the requirements of study. Image scaling, background removal, noise reduction, augmentation, and other processes are among them.

3. Image Segmentation: To find contaminated patches in photos, image segmentation is used. Segmentation aids in identifying just the aspects of an image that are important to the task at hand.

4. Features Extraction: The feature extraction procedure detects the main distinguishing properties of chosen items in the picture. The image processing approach is commonly used to extract features from pictures. Deep neural networks, on the other hand, now play a key part in automated feature extraction from image samples. Relevant characteristics are often extracted from pictures by extracting colour, shape, and texture-related attributes from an area of interest (AOI). To categorise a given picture sample into a certain class label, a classification approach is utilised.

5. Disease classification: ML algorithms are utilized to design and develop ML classifiers. Extracted features are fed as input into machine learning models to perform classification task. Diseases are categorized by using trained ML models.

In our work, we have applied deep learning approach using deep CNN architecture in place of traditional machine learning approach to eliminate the use of image processing-based feature extraction module. Deep CNN approach combines features extraction and disease classification in one unit. This approach not only reduces processing time but also increases the recognition and classification accuracy of the system due to deep learning of the features. Many times, researchers apply CNN only for learning of the features, then learned features are fed into machine learning models to recognise and categorize the diseases.

Deep CNN architecture learns the significant features so deeply and nicely that it gives promising result even for unprocessed input data. In fact, above discussed image pre-processing and segmentation modules are optional in deep learning model for plant disease diagnosis. But researchers keep using these two modules according to the requirement of the problem domain. In this work we have focussed our study on 3 types of deadly rice diseases namely; Leaf smut, bacterial blight, and brown spot.

Samples of these diseases are shown in Figure 3.2, Figure 3.3 and Figure 3.4 respectively. Symptoms and appearance of these diseases are discussed in chapter 1 (under section 1.5.1).

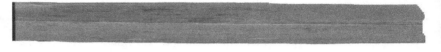

Figure 3.2 Sample of Leaf smut infection [97]

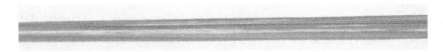

Figure 3.3 Sample of Bacterial Leaf Blight infection [97]

Figure 3.4 Sample of Brown spot infection [97]

3.2 Related work

To diagnose tomato plant leaf illnesses, Atabay (2017) [86] used 4 different CNN models on the PlantVillage database. VGG19 and VGG16, the first two structures, are pre-trained networks, whereas the other two are suggested customised networks. To acquire a residual CNN architecture, the suggested CNN architecture was given training with residual learning, whereas to get a simple CNN structure, the suggested CNN architecture was trained without residual learning. After analysing the performance of all 4 architectures, it was discovered that the residual CNN architecture outperforms the other three. The residual CNN model was 97.53 percent accurate.

Liang et al. (2019) [87] created a new CNN-based method for detecting rice blast illness. Plant protection specialists provided them with 2906 diseased and 2902 healthy images of rice leaf. To extract distinguishing characteristics from input image, local binary patterns histograms, Wavelet transform, and CNN were utilised. SVM used these characteristics to categorise the blast illness. The CNN provides selected and more significant features than the other 2 approaches. According to the results analysis, the accuracy of SVM with CNN was 95.82 percent, whereas the accuracy of SVM with LBPH was 82.59 percent.

A similar approach was used by Bodapati et al. (2019) [54] to extract features automatically from the images. Authors have designed a DCNN architecture to capture the most significant characteristics from the input sample. Three CL and PL are followed by a fully connected output layer in this design. The receptive field of the first CL was a 5 * 5 block, and each picture was made up of numerous blocks that were overlapping. As a result, each picture was characterized by 28*28 overlapping receptive fields. A CL was made up of many feature maps; in this case, the first CL has six feature maps. To decrease the number of parameters to be calculated, the weights of all neurons of the same feature map were kept similar.

After obtaining the features, they conducted 2 experiments to categorize the diseases. In the first experiment, ANN with 2 hidden layers was utilized to perform the classification of illnesses. In the second experiment, SVM was used to categorize the diseases. The accuracy of SVM as a classifier utilizing DCNN features was approximately identical or slightly better than that of ANN as a classifier.

Kumbhar et al. (2019) [88] developed a CNN-based cotton disease classification system. A cotton leaf picture was collected from a benchmarked dataset to provide training to the classifier. 720 cotton leaf photos were obtained from dataset, in which 513 pictures were used to train the model and 207 leaves pictures were used to validate the model. Python programming environment was used to implement CNN. CNN is made up of 3 convolution layers, each convolution layer is followed by ReLU and Max pooling layers. Each CL contained 64 distinct filters to capture the features. Size of convolving window was 3*3 with stride size as 4. To pick the maximum probability, the Softmax layer linearizes the illness probabilities in a single dimensional matrix. On training dataset, the suggested model was 80% accurate, while on test dataset, it had an accuracy of 89 percent.

Tahir et al. (2018) [89] present a new fungus database for detecting and distinguishing various forms of fungus using CNN. Authors have collected fungal spores images from infected fruits. Suggested new data set consisted of 40,800 pictures of fungal spores. These images contained 5 varieties of fungal spores. With 5-fold validation, the developed CNN model achieved 94.8 percent accuracy.

3.3 Methods and Materials

We have proposed two approaches for diagnosis and classification of rice diseases. The suggested approaches for rice leaf illness diagnosis and classification are described in this section. Image samples acquisition from dataset collection, pre-processing of collected pictures, designing of effective CNN architecture to capture significant features, and disease classification are the key processes illustrated in both approaches. Both approaches utilized same deep CNN architecture. Flow diagram of suggested work is depicted in Figure 3.5.

3.3.1 Basic steps used in proposed work

The following are the basic processes involved in suggested work:

1. Image Acquisition: This is very first step in DIP applications. The process of collecting the required input picture samples for further analysis is known as image acquisition.

2. Image pre-processing: Pre-processing is an important step in obtaining a high-quality image and assuring the accuracy of the image's attributes. The key pre-processing operations covered in this step are image size reduction, leaf area segmentation by removing complex background information, and cropping.

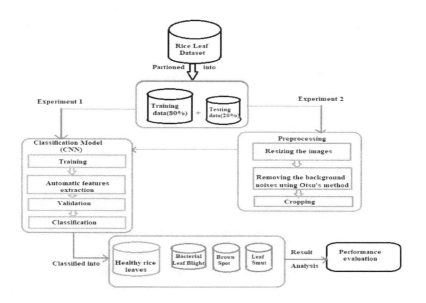

Figure 3.5 Flow diagram of Proposed Work

3. Automatic features extraction: A series of repeated Convolution and pooling layers of DCNN [54] with the different number of filters is designed to extract the characteristics of pictures automatically. Dimension of filters kept different at different convolution layer.

4. Classification of diseases: To categorise the plant diseases, the DCNN model uses a fully connected layer followed by a softmax layer as the final layer. The Softmax layer linearizes the sickness probabilities in a single dimensional matrix to determine the maximum probability corresponding to a particular disease. Disease with maximum probability is depicted as output class.

A convolution neural network completes the automatic feature extraction and illness classification operations in one unit. The above outlined steps are covered in further depth in the next subsequent subsections for both approaches.

58

3.3.2 First proposed approach

In this approach, unprocessed leaf picture samples acquired from dataset are directly given to the proposed deep CNN architecture for features extraction. Here in this approach no pre-processing operation is performed on input samples. Whole image with background information is processed by the suggested deep CNN architecture.

3.3.2.1 Data set description

In order to conduct the two suggested investigations, we used a rice leaf database. The dataset is made up of four different varieties of rice leaves picture samples accessed from Kaggle [90]. As indicated in Table 3.1, each variety of rice leaves is made up of 4000 rice leaves pictures. These are photographs of both sick and healthy leaves. Among four classes, three classes belong to diseased leaves and one class belongs to healthy leaves. In these three classes, one class consists of Brown Spot infected leaves images, the second class consists of Bacterial Leaf Blight infected leaves images, and the third class contains Leaf Smut infected leaves images. Figure 3.6 depicts a healthy and sick sample of rice leaf pictures adopted in this study.

Table 3.1 Description of Dataset

Paddy leaf Classes	Samples count
Bacterial Leaf Blight (BLB)	4,000
Leaf Smut (LS)	4,000
Brown Spot (BS)	4,000
Healthy Leaves	4,000

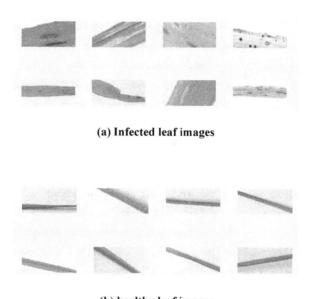

(a) Infected leaf images

(b) healthy leaf images

Figure 3.6   Dataset samples (a) Infected leaf images (b) healthy leaf images

3.3.2.2 Data Pre-processing

Only image resizing pre-processing operation is performed in first approach. First approach is developed without removing the background information from picture samples. Whole image with background is given as input to the proposed system.

3.3.2.3 Designing of deep CNN architecture for automatic features extraction and classification

To categorize the rice illnesses and improve the precision and efficiency of our approach, we used the convolution neural network (CNN) architecture. CNN outperforms classical learning approaches, and it's commonly employed in variety of computer vision applications. Numerous hidden layers are utilized to assess and refine the most relevant attributes of the input samples, input samples are provided to the network by an input layer, and an output layer is placed to deliver the network output. These layers are utilised to carry out numerous tasks required to complete the given task. The number of hidden layers changes according to the situation and is determined by the nature of the problem. Convolution and pooling operations are the key operations performed in hidden layers to extract the significant image attributes required for image classification. Fully connected layers are placed at final position of CNN to perform classification task.

The CL, which performs the required number of the convolution operations, involving features learning, is a key component of CNN. Biases, padding, the size of the kernels, the value of the stride, and number of kernels are used in convolution operations Liu et al. (2018) [91] to learn the features. The number of pixels by which a fixed-size filter slides on input data is called stride. A filter is another name for a kernel. Filter are two-dimensional matrices which sizes always maintained shorter than the input picture size. Figure 3.7 discussed by Phung et al. (2018) [92] depicts the basic structure of CNN.

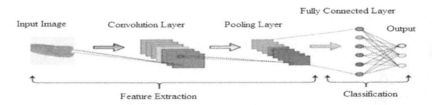

Figure 3.7 Basic structure of CNN [92]

The CL takes an input picture and transforms it by convolving it with a filter. The CL generates a number of feature maps for an input picture. When a fixed size filter is applied to a picture, the summation of pixel values respective to the filter's values is computed.

As a result of this calculation, multiple feature maps (corresponding to different filters) are generated for the given picture. A collection of several CL with different filter sizes might be used to recognise complicated characteristics. As input moves further into the deeper layer in network, we have used a common strategy of

61

increasing the number of filters and decreasing their dimensions. Equation (3.1) Liu et al. (2018) [56] is used to compute the transformation operation by convolution layer.

$$O_n^l = \left(\sum_{m \in X_n} O_m^{l-1} * F_{mn}^l + B_n^l \right) \qquad (3.1)$$

where, lth layer's convolution output is represented by O_n^l and (l-1) th layer's convolution output is represented by O_m^{l-1}. F_{mn}^l represents convolution filter of lth layer and B_n^l represents lth layer's bias. Selection of input map is represented by Xn.

After the CL, the ReLU layer is utilized to convert all negative values of feature maps to zero. ReLU is recommended as an activation function because of its ability to quickly converge. Equation (3.2) used by Bodapati et al. (2019) [54] shows how to compute the activation function.

$$Activation(input) = maximum(0, input) \qquad (3.2)$$

The ReLU layer's output is then sent to the max-pooling layer, which determines the highest values of the pixels in a particular pool size. The downsampling layer is another name of the pooling layer. The downsampling layers do not change the amount of feature maps; instead, it changes the size of the features as discussed by Zhu et al. (2018) [94]. The Max-pooling layer uses the sampling mask to minimise the dimensions of feature maps. As a result, the pooling layer decreases the number of characteristics that must be learned.

Four CLs are employed in the suggested network to extract significant characteristics from the dataset's pictures. Each input channel is normalized using a batch normalization layer (BNL) across a mini-batch size. BNL is used just after the Convolution layer (CL). BNL is followed by the ReLu layer. The ReLu layer removes the negative activations. After the ReLu layer, the max-pool layer is utilized to select the most significant features of the feature map. thus max-pooling layer down-samples the input picture. The network's last layer is made up of 4 FC layers (flatten layers) along with a Softmax layer that divides the pictures into 4 categories (1 healthy and 3 sick). A feed-forward neural network is employed to perform the classification operation at the FC layer. The structure of the proposed CNN is shown in Table 3.2.

First model is developed without removing the background information from picture samples. Whole image with background is given as input to the proposed system. In first model, only image resizing operation is used as pre-processing step.

Table 3.2 Structure of proposed fully connected CNN

S.N.	Layer's type	Filter's size and Strides	Input size	Learnables
1.	Input	64 x 64 x 3	64x64x3	-
2.	CL	8 9x9x3/1	64x64x8	Weights 9x9x3x8 Bias 1x1x8
3.	BNL	Batch-Normalization with eight channels	64x64x8	Offset 1x1x8 Scale 1x1x8
4.	RL	ReLU	64x64x8	-
5.	MPL	2x2/2	32x32x8	-
6.	CL	16 6x6x8/1	32x32x16	Weights 6x6x8x16 Bias 1x1x8
7.	BNL	Batch-Normalization with sixteen channels	32x32x16	Offset 1x1x16 Scale 1x1x16
8.	RL	ReLU	32x32x16	-
9.	MPL	2x2/2	16x16x16	-
10.	CL	32 3x3x16/1	16x16x32	Weights 3x3x16x32 Bias 1x1x32
11.	BNL	Batch-Normalization with thirty-two channels	16x16x32	Offset 1x1x32 Scale 1x1x32
12.	RL	ReLU	16x16x32	-
13.	MPL	2x2/2	8x8x32	-
14.	CL	64 3x3x32/1	8x8x64	Weights 3x3x32x64 Bias 1x1x64
15.	BNL	Batch-Normalization with sixty-four channels	8x8x64	Offset 1x1x64 Scale 1x1x64
16.	RL	ReLU	8x8x64	-

17.	FC	4 FC layers	1x1x4	Weights 4x4096 Bias 4x1
18.	Softmax Layer	Softmax	1x1x4	-
19.	Classification Output	Classification	-	-

3.3.3 Second proposed approach

In this approach, processed leaf picture samples are given to the same proposed deep CNN architecture for features extraction. Here, in this approach image pre-processing is performed on input samples to remove the background information.

3.3.3.1 Data set description

Same dataset as discussed in approach 1 is utilized here to acquire leaf image samples of rice plant to provide input to the image pre-processing module.

3.3.3.2 Image pre-processing

Image size reduction, leaf area segmentation by removing complex background information, and cropping techniques are all part of the pre-processing step. To begin pre-processing, a resizing operation is performed on input picture samples to produce resized pictures of 64 *64 dimensions. The second step in picture pre-processing is background information elimination to get leaf part from the image. To remove the background, each RGB picture is converted to a blue color picture by setting the red and green elements to zero. The mean values of green, blue and red elements are then

used to turn each blue channel picture into a grayscale image. Figure 3.8 shows a grayscale representation of an example rice leaf picture.

To construct a binary mask, the Otsu technique is now applied to the grayscale picture. To conduct picture binarization, Otsu global thresholding approach is used. The between-class variance (or within-class variance) depending on a picture histogram is calculated and evaluated in this thresholding approach to discover all possible threshold values. The optimal threshold value is determined by recording the threshold corresponding to the maximum between-class variation (or minimal within-class variance). After determining the best threshold value, all picture elements with intensity smaller than the threshold are assigned with zero values, while the intensities of other pixels are turned to 1. As a result, the thresholding operation produces a binary mask for the grey picture. A binary mask picture is one in which each picture element has a value of zero or non-zero. Picture element with zero value indicates that the picture element belongs to background, whereas picture element with non-zero value belong to the foreground (area of interest). Figure 3.9 illustrates the binary mask created by Otsu's approach [95] on a sample grayscale picture. The region of interest is created by multiplying this binary mask with the original picture. Figure 3.10 depicts an example picture after removal of background. Image cropping is the final stage in the image pre-processing process. Cropping a photograph improves its visual appearance even further.

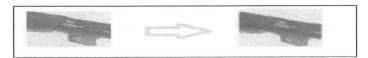

Figure. 3.8 Transformation of RGB image into Grayscale Image

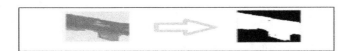

Figure 3.9 Creation of Binary mask from gray scale image

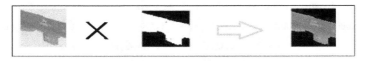

Figure 3.10 Background removal

3.3.3.3 Extraction of features and classification

We have utilized same deep CNN architecture as discussed in approach 1 to learn the relevant image attributes automatically. FC layers placed at final position of the network use these extracted features to complete the classification process. Softmax layer is used just after FC layers to compute classification probability of input instance. During the learning process of the model, cross-entropy loss is used as a cost function to alter the network's weights.

3.4 Implementation and Results

The experimental setting and performance analysis of the suggested plant disease diagnosis and classification technique are discussed in this section. Training and validation datasets, hardware descriptions, and software details are illustrated in the experimental environment. Total 2 experiments are conducted: one for approach 1 and other for approach 2. Experiment related to approach 1 is named as Experiment 1 while experiment related to approach 2 is named as Experiment 2. Further, the training and validation process of approach 1, the validation and training process of approach 2, the contrast of results of approach 1 and approach 2, and finally a comparative study of the suggested method with some prior works are all included in this section. All discussions are organized in 5 subsections.

3.4.1 Experimental environment

The dataset with picture of rice leaves is obtained via Kaggle [90]. There are three categories of sick leaves in this dataset, as well as one category of healthy leaves. On this dataset, we have conducted two experiments for the two approaches: the first experiment is related to the implementation of a deep CNN model without background removal from input samples, and the second experiment deals with the implementation of a deep CNN model with background removal from input samples using Otsu's global thresholding technique. The dataset is partitioned into 80:20 partitions, with 80 percent serving as a training dataset and 20 percent serving as a testing dataset to validate the model. All of the experiments are run on a DELL laptop with a Core i5 CPU running at 1.80 GHz. The memory capacity of the above said laptop is four GB DDRAM with 250 GB SSD. This laptop is equipped with Windows 10 OS. In implementation, all the experiments are performed in MATLAB R2019a.

3.4.2 Training-validation observation of approach 1 (experiment 1)

Experiment 1 was carried out by feeding the suggested deep CNN model with original data. Here, we have evaluated the suggested model's classification performance for approach 1. The model's training and validation were experimented using the training-validation samples listed in Table 3.3. We used eight epochs, each of which had 100 iterations. To observe the results of approach 1(experiment 1), a total of 800 iterations were performed. Training process and Validation steps are illustrated in figure 3.11a. Here, Figure 3.11a depicts model's accuracy vs. the number of epochs during training-validation process.

Table 3.3 Training-Validation sample counts

Leaves Categories	Total images	Training Image counts	Validation Image counts
Healthy	4,000	3,200	800
Brown spot	4,000	3,200	800
Bacterial leaf blight	4,000	3,200	800
Leaf smut	4,000	3,200	800

Figure 3.11b shows the changes in loss as the number of epochs increases. For validation and training datasets, Loss interprets model goodness. A model with a smaller loss is a better model. The model's performance is depicted using a confusion matrix. The suggested model's right and wrong classifications for approach 1 are depicted in Figure. 3.12 using a confusion matrix. Here, predicted disease is shown along y axis whereas actual disease is shown along x-axis in confusion matrix.

The recalls of the individual class are depicted at lower most row in confusion matrix. The precision of the individual disease category is depicted in the rightmost-column of the confusion matrix. The overall accuracy of the developed system is indicated by the rightmost-bottom cell, which represents the average accuracy of the suggested disease classifier for approach 1(experiment 1).

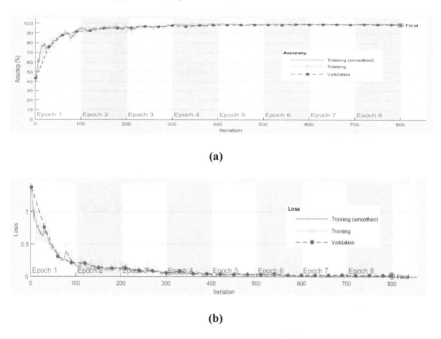

(a)

(b)

Figure 3.11 (a) Training-validation accuracy of model using Experiment1, (b) Training-validation Loss-rate of model using Experiment1

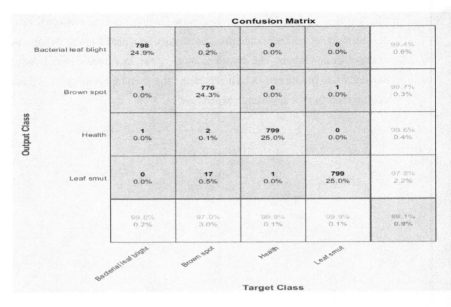

Figure 3.12 Classification result using Confusion matrix (Experiment1)

3.4.3 Training-validation observation of approach 2 (experiment 2)

The developed deep CNN architecture is utilized in approach 2(experiment 2) using a pre-processed dataset. Background information from each and every sample image is removed via pre-processing. To eliminate the background from the leaf picture, a global thresholding approach proposed by Otsu is utilized. The suggested model's classification results for approach 2 were examined in this section. The processed dataset with the same training and validation division as shown in Table 3.3. is used to train and validate the proposed model. The same number of epochs, as well as the same number of iterations per epoch as discussed in approach 1, is used to provide learning to the suggested system. Both studies use the same training and validation setup. The validation and training accuracy of the proposed system for approach 2 during the validation and training process is depicted in Figure 3.13a, while the loss observed in validation and training is depicted in Figure 3.13b. The frequency of validation is set at 30 iterations. With the use of a confusion matrix, right and wrong predictions of the suggested deep CNN architecture for approach 2 have displayed in Figure. 3.14. The background removed images improves the learning ability of the suggested model, resulting in an increase in accuracy from 99.1 percent to 99.7 percent and a decrease in the loss with the equivalent proportion. Although this improvement in accuracy is not much, but in the case of complex background, more improvement in accuracy can be achieved by using second approach.

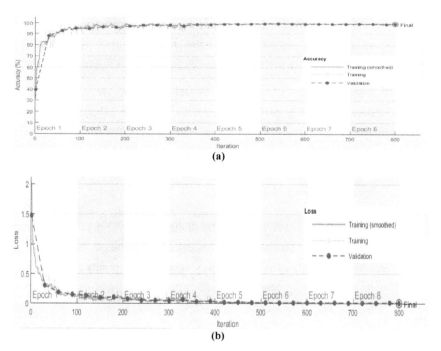

Figure 3.13 (a) Training-validation accuracy of model using Experiment2, (b) Training-validation Loss-rate of model using Experiment2

The model with pre-processed data can now learn the discriminating characteristics of images in such a good manner that erroneous classification is reduced to zero in leaf smut and healthy classes, and minimized to 1.2 percent in brown spot and 0.1 percent in bacterial leaf blight (BLB) cases. One BLB-infected picture out of 800 is incorrectly labeled as a brown spot, whereas ten brown spot-infected photos are incorrectly categorized as leaf smut.

3.4.4 Results contrast between approach 1 and approach 2

In approach 1, two BLB-diseased leaves out of 800 are misclassified, one as healthy and the other as brown spot, but just one BLB leaf is misclassified in approach 2. In approach 1, a total of 24 samples out of 800 brown spot affected leaves are wrongly labeled in which five samples are misclassified as BLB, seventeen are misclassified as leaf smut, and 2 samples are misclassified as healthy. But only ten samples of the brown spot are wrongly categorized as leaf smut in approach 2.

In approach 1, one healthy leaf and one leaf smut image are incorrectly categorized, while in approach 2, no leaf is incorrectly labeled in either healthy or leaf smut situations. The suggested architecture with approach 2 conducts the learning more properly and accurately and hence diagnoses the rice plant illness more correctly, as shown by the analysis of the results. Approach 1 and approach 2 accuracies are compared in Figure 3.15.

3.4.5 Results comparison of proposed approaches with the existing techniques

We compared the accuracy of our suggested approaches to that of other previous leaf disease classification and diagnosis methods. The comparison of our suggested model with existing methods is based on the frequent practice of recognizing and identifying plant diseases using photographs of plant leaves.

To identify plant illness, all of the methods compared here utilized images of plant leaf samples. The majority of the approaches used in this comparison have utilized deep CNN architectures for disease detection.

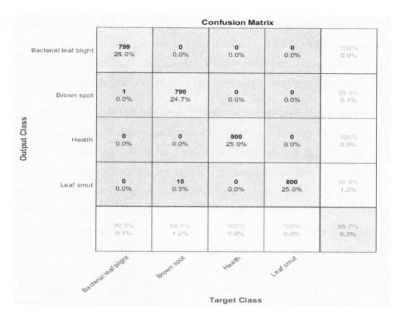

Figure 3.14 Classification result using Confusion matrix (Experiment2)

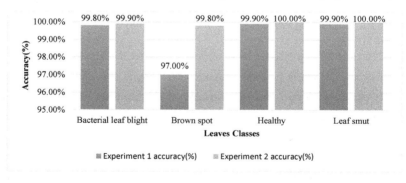

Figure 3.15 Accuracies contrast of Approach 1 and Approach 2

SVM-based model, SVM oriented prediction model using K-means segmentation, CNN based classifier, SVM classifier with CNN based features extraction, residual CNN model, GoogleNet CNN architecture, AlexNet deep learning, and SqueezeNet deep learning were used to compare findings of our approaches. Soybean, cotton, tomato, and Rice are the plants included in this comparative study. Our suggested approaches outperformed other current approaches, according to our findings. Figure 3.16 shows a comparison of past approaches' accuracy with our approaches.

The suggested approaches can effectively analyze large datasets and do not require separate feature extraction modules, which is not possible with traditional approaches. The main issue is that we would need high-speed GPUs to handle these enormous datasets. Many present approaches struggle to extract the most important feature because in these approaches feature extraction requires manual intervention. Our solution solves this challenge by automatically extracting features. Automatic feature extraction is employed in few of the current approaches addressed in the literature review (Liang et al. (2019) [87], Kumbhar et al. [88], Jadhav et al. (2020) [75]), however, our suggested methodology outperforms these methods due to effective deep CNN architecture and superior background elimination approach. In our technique, Otsu's thresholding method aids in the recognition of plant leaves from their surroundings.

3.5 Concluding remarks

This research provided a novel method for detecting and categorizing illnesses found in rice plants by combining 4 hidden layered CNN with Otsu's thresholding-based background removal strategy. This method extracts distinguishing characteristics from leaf pictures based on the color, shape, and size of infected regions in the leaves. Deep CNN architecture is designed so well that it is able to recognize and categorize rice diseases with great accuracy (99.10%). From the validation and training process depicted in experiment 1 (Figure 3.11), it is very clear that the suggested approach 1 does not face an overfitting problem.

This is due to the efficient tunning of the proposed model and the availability of a large dataset. In approach 2, to focus only on the leaf portion in input sample, pre-processing is conducted to the input sample to eliminate background information. The suggested approaches decrease model complexity as well as processing time by combining feature extraction and disease categorization into a single CNN unit, while also improving classification results.

S.No.	Authors	Methods	Plant	Accuracy
1	Prajapati et al. (2017) [51]	SVM based predictive model with K-means clustering segmentation	Rice	73.33%
2	Atabay et al. (2017) [86]	Residual CNN model	Tomato	97.53%
3	Liang et al. (2019) [87]	CNN to extract features and SVM as classifier	Rice	95.82%
4	Liang et al. (2019) [87]	LBPH to extract features and SVM as classifier	Rice	82.59%
5	Kumbhar et al.(2019)[88]	CNN based classifier	Cotton	89%
6	Sanjay Patidar et al. (2020) [64]	Residual neural network	Rice	95.83%
7	Sachin et al. (2020) [75]	GoogleNet CNN architecture	Soybean	96.25%
8	Sachin et al. (2020) [75]	AlexNet	Soybean	98.75%
9	**Upadhyay and Kumar [7]**	Proposed CNN based classifier	Rice	99.10%
10	**Upadhyay and Kumar [7]**	Proposed CNN based classifier with Otsu's method	Rice	99.70%

Figure 3.16 Comparative analysis of accuracies of proposed model with existing models

Both approaches performed admirably, according to our findings. The initial model, which did not use background removal, learned the distinguishing traits so well that it achieved a 99.1% accuracy rate. The second approach with background elimination outperforms the first approach with an accuracy of 99.7 percent, according to the analysis of the results. Our models' performance was compared to that of existing approaches, and our models were determined to be highly adequate.

CHAPTER 4

EARLY-STAGE BROWN SPOT DISEASES DIAGNOSIS IN PADDY CROP USING IMAGE PROCESSING AND DEEP CNN ARCHITECTURE

4.1 Introduction

Crop yields have a big influence on both domestic and international financial systems. Agriculture is extremely important to India's economy. Crop development is heavily influenced by biological and climatic variables. Plant diseases are one of the key biological variables that, if not diagnosed and managed in a timely manner, can great loss to crop production. In precision agriculture, plant disease diagnosis and classification are very important and essential procedures as talked by Gavhale et al. (2014) [96]. Disease detection is still mostly done by physical examination with the bare eyes. It is quite hard for professionals to regularly monitor big fields. Physical examination with the bare eyes might be inaccurate and ineffective. Therefore, it is extremely beneficial if the rice crop illness is automatically diagnosed in a timely manner. Farmers will be benefited greatly from the adoption of computerized disease diagnosis and recognition as suggested by Kulkarni et al. (2012) [40].

This chapter focuses on fungus-caused brown spot illness found in paddy crops. This is such a serious infection that it can cause up to 50% yield loss when it becomes intense. The brown spot starts out as tiny dots of brown color, then grows into an oval to circular, or tubular shape. Brown spot has a high likelihood of spreading and growing in the soils which have a deficiency of nutrients and micronutrients. A Brown spot usually damages the plant's leaves, grains, and stems. The Helminthosporium oryzae organism causes it, and it damages the plant from seed germination to the milky stage. Figure 2 shows a brown spot infected rice leaf sample.

75

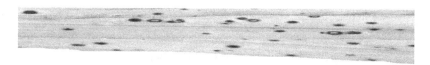

Figure 4.1 Brown spot diseased rice leaf [97]

Generally, it is noticed that the essential building blocks of any crop disease diagnosis system include both machine learning and digital image processing. Figure 1 depicted in previous chapter 3 is a generic method to plant disease diagnosis using DIP and ML techniques.

In this thesis, we have proposed brown spot disease diagnosis method for rice crop that is able to capture this disease at very initial stage. This type of approach is beneficial for the farmers, since spread of disease can be stopped at initial stage by applying appropriate treatment procedures. We have used DIP techniques to label the brown spot disease based on infection severity. Further, Deep CNN architecture is developed to build early-stage brown spot disease diagnosis model.

4.1.1 Motivation

Farmers can use a plant disease diagnosis system to identify and classify crop diseases correctly. After an accurate diagnosis of crop diseases, farmers can apply suitable preventive measures to treat the crops. Many researchers have developed several crop disease diagnosis methods, but very few of them proposed disease diagnosis based on disease severity computation. Most researchers have classified the diseases based on their types and name. Such types of classifications are not sufficient, since it does not give any indication about the appropriate quantity of pesticide that can be used in the treatment of the diseases. If pesticide/insecticide is not applied in an appropriate quantity, it fails to treat the diseases properly. If an overdose of pesticide is used then it causes soil pollution, wastage of money, and even damage to the crops. On the other hand, if an underdose of pesticide is used then it cannot cure the diseases properly. Therefore, it is required that a proper quantity of fertilizers and pesticides should be used in plant disease treatment. To address these types of issues, we have proposed a disease diagnosis and classification method based on infection severity estimation. Our approach is able to diagnose and classify the paddy disease at an early stage. So, by applying proper preventive measures at the initial stage, the further spread can be stopped. Further, our approach is able to categorize the disease into one of the 3 categories: healthy, early-stage, and developed stage. This type of classification assists the farmers to decide the proper quantity of insecticide to treat the crop infections.

4.1.2 Research Objectives

The major goal of this chapter is to identify the brown spot illness in rice crop at very initial stage so that losses can be avoided. The objective may be broken down into the following tasks:

1. Investigating the limitations of the most effective methods for plant leaf disease detection and severity estimation approaches which were reviewed in chapter 2.

2. DIP techniques are employed in the suggested work to locate and segment the lesions and to estimate the infection severity in rice leaf image samples.

3. Derivation of infection severity-based disease classes for acquired brown spot disease.

4. Developing a novel automated deep learning approach to detect deadly brown spot disease at very early-stage.

5. Enhancing detection accuracy and reducing the mistake rate by using proposed deep CNN architecture

4.1.3 Organization of the Chapter

Remaining of this chapter comprise of the following sections:
Section 2 In this section some related works are discussed.

Section 3 This section discusses materials and methods used in proposed "Early-stage brown spot disease detection model".

Section 4 This section discusses implementation and results of the proposed model.

Section 5 This Section provide summery of the proposed work.

4.2 Related Work

In this section, we discuss about some reviewed effective methods used for infection severity estimation.

Powbunthorn et al. (2012) [98] suggested a technique for determining the degree of illness (severity) in cassava crops. This paper focused on brown spot illness. They first convert the RGB picture into an HSI format. The sick picture elements are obtained after this transformation by isolating the Hue component. Furthermore, the ratio of area of infected region to area of total leaf region was used to compute the severity of infection. Area of infected regions was represented by the number of pixels present in infected regions.

A technique to measure the intensity of infection found on rice leaves was provided by Islam et al. (2015) [99]. To get diseased and healthy leaves clusters, the K-Means algorithm was used to the input leaf picture. To compute the pixels count in the healthy area, a segmented picture with a healthy component was transformed into a binary picture. To determine the pixels count in the infected section, a Segmented picture with a diseased component was transformed into a binary picture. The sample leaf's total number of pixels was then determined as the sum of diseased and healthy pixel counts. Ultimately, the ratio of diseased pixel number to total leaf pixel number was used to determine the disease severity of the sample leaf image.

With the goal of providing the intensity of disease, Patil et al. (2011) [100] conducted research on evaluating the severity of sugar cane leaf disease by applying 2 phase segmentation approach. In first segmentation, simple thresholding was used to identify the leaf region. In second level segmentation, infected regions were recognised using triangle thresholding on transformed HSI pictures. The proportion of

78

the diseased area to the leaf area was used to determine the disease severity. The accuracy of the results was found to be 98.60 percent.

BLSNet, a new technique for Rice BLS disease detection and severity assessment, was developed by Chen et al. (2021) [101]. BLSNet is a deep learning network that employs the semantic segmentation idea. To improve the accuracy of illness segmentation, the suggested model included multi-scale extraction and an attention mechanism. The authors trained the proposed network using actual photographs of paddy fields. The effectiveness of the BLSNet was contrasted against DeepLabv3+ and UNet, two deep learning networks with semantic segmentation. According to the authors, the suggested model outperformed the others in terms of segmentation and classification accuracy.

Liang et al. (2019) [102] suggested a deep CNN-based model for plant illness diagnosis and severity estimation. To generate a greater number of samples, the Augmentation technique was utilized. By using augmentation large dataset was created, and training with this large dataset minimizes the overfitting problem of the suggested network. This model is named as PD2SE-Net by the authors. Here ResNet50 architecture was utilized as a base model to develop the suggested network. To generate shuffle architecture in the network, ShuffleNet-V2 was utilized. Thus, the proposed model was developed by combining the ResNet50 and ShuffleNet-V2 architectures. Along with illness detection and severity estimation, the proposed model is also able to identify the species of plants. In result analysis, disease detection and severity estimation accuracies were observed as 98 % and 91%, respectively. Whereas species of plants were recognized with 99% accuracy.

4.3. Methods And Materials

This section describes the dataset and acquisition of brown spot images from the dataset. Next, infection severity estimation is described using two-phase segmentations. Further, the creation of a new derived dataset using estimated infection severity is illustrated. Finally, Deep Convolution architecture and its work to extract the features and classify the early-stage infection are discussed. These methods and materials are presented in different subsections.

4.3.1 Dataset

The dataset for paddy leaves was obtained from Kaggle [90]. There are four different types of rice leaves organized in 4 different classes in this dataset. Each class contains 4000 leaf photographs. One class consists of all leaf images of brown spot (BS) disease. The other 3 classes consist of all images of BLB disease, Leaf Smut (LS) disease, and healthy leaves, respectively. Each class of the dataset is shown in Table 3.1 (chapter 3). Figure 3.6 shows sample photos of diseased and normal leaves acquired from the dataset. In the suggested work, we have selected very common and deadly paddy disease known as brown spot for the study.

4.3.2 Basic steps used in proposed work

The basic steps used in proposed work are given below:

1. Acquisition of healthy and brown spot infected leaf samples: The healthy leaf samples and brown spot leaf samples are chosen from the paddy leaves database [90]. These two types of samples are used for further processing in our work.

2. Estimation of infection severity and partition of collected brown spot class: The following basic sub-steps are required for this process:

(a) Leaf area segmentation from brown spot picture samples

(b) Infected area segmentation from segmented leaf area

(c) Infection severity computation

(d) Partitioning of collected brown spot infected class into developed stage Brown spot(DSBS) class and early-stage brown spot(ESBS) class based on computed severity of each and every infected leaf.

3. Automatic Features Extraction: To extract the relevant discriminating features of DSBS samples, ESBS samples and healthy leaf samples, a CNN based effective and simple architecture comprising of various serial combinations of CL and PL was developed.

4. Recognition of brown spot at Initial stage: The suggested CNN architecture's final layer is a FC layer backed by a SoftMax layer. The final layer is utilised to determine if the given leaf sample has initial level infection or developed infection or no infection at all.

The steps indicated above are explored in more detail in the following subsections. A flow diagram depicting the suggested strategy for diagnosing and classifying Brown spot disease at the initial level in paddy plants is depicted in Figure 4.2.

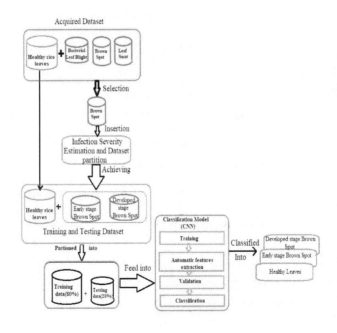

Figure 4.2 Flow diagram of suggested method

4.3.3 Estimation of Severity of Infection (IS) and Partition of collected Brown spot dataset

In this phase, each and every brown spot infected leaf picture are segmented twice in a serial way. To locate the leaf area in the input picture, the segmentation1 is performed using thresholding(global) approach suggested by Otsu. During segmentation2 process, the infected regions are obtained by applying triangle thresholding to the segmented leaf region. Pixel counts in infected area and total pixel counts in the complete leaf area are calculated separately. Eq. 4.1 is used to compute the infection severity (IS) :

$$\text{Infection severity (IS)} = N1 / N2 \qquad\qquad (4.1)$$

Where N1 is pixel counts in infected area N2 is pixel counts in entire Leaf area.

Brown spot infected leaf pictures are either included in the DSBS class or in the ESBS class, depending on computed severity of the infection. Together with healthy leaf samples, these two generated classes form a new derived database for the Early-stage illness recognition model. In algorithm 1, which is structured in sub-section 4.3.3.4 and shown in Figure 4.11, the details of Infection Severity calculation process as well as dataset splitting approach are presented. Figure 4.3 depicts the flow diagram for this approach.

4.3.3.1 Image Acquisition of Brown Spots

In this work, Brown spot leaf pictures are selected from the paddy leaves database [90] for the investigation. By deleting redundant and dull photos from 4,000 brown spot photographs, only 3,008 excellent quality pictures are obtained. We created two new classes based on obtained brown-spot pictures: ESBS and DSBS. The suggested early-stage brown-spot illness recognition model is tested using these freshly created classes, as well as 4,000 healthy leaf samples taken from the paddy leaves database.

82

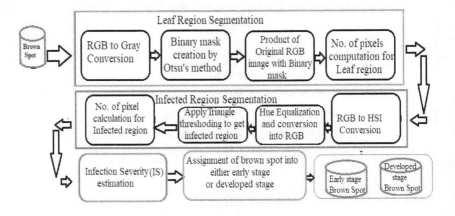

Figure 4.3 Estimation of Severity of Infection (IS) and Partition of collected Brown spot dataset

4.3.3.2 Segmentation of Leaf Region

The photos are resized to 64*64 dimensions using DIP operation. The image transformation process is used to transform a RGB picture into a Gray-scale picture. Figure 4.4 shows a sample Gray-scale picture transformed from a RGB image. The global thresholding approach of Otsu (1979) [95] is used to create the binary mask. The Gray-scale picture is first transformed into a picture histogram. Then, the histogram is used to compute and evaluate the with-in-class variance by Otsu's method to find all potential thresholds. The best threshold is chosen based on the smallest with-in-class variance. Picture elements with values below the computed threshold are set as 0, while the rest picture element's values are changed to 1. Picture elements with values of 0 form the background, whereas picture elements with values of 1 form the leaf-region (foreground). A binary mask is created with picture elements that have 0 or 1 values. To eliminate noisy artifacts from the binary image, a flood-fill process is used. Figure 4.5 shows the binary mask of an example Gray-scale picture. To create a segmented leaf section of a given RGB image, the computed binary mask is multiplied by the original RGB picture. Figure 4.6 depicts the leaf area segmented by this procedure.

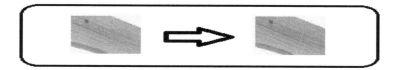

Figure 4.4 Grayscale converted image of a RGB image

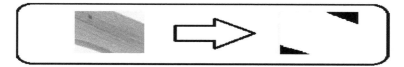

Figure 4.5 Conversion of Grayscale image into Binary image

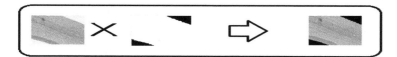

Figure 4.6 Segmentation of Leaf part from input sample

4.3.3.3 Segmentation of Diseased Areas

Appropriate DIP techniques are required to identify the correct infected area in the leaf. Accurate segmentation of the diseased areas is required for further effective experimentation outcomes. Because the lesion is faded in color in the initial stages of the illness, therefore segmentation findings may be poor. Lesions express distinct symptoms at different phases of the illness due to the influence of multiple environmental elements such as light and water. The segmentation is adversely affected by this circumstance. To prevent these problems, the segmented RGB picture produced by the first segmentation is first transformed into an HSI picture, which is a more human-friendly visual system. The hue element has been discovered to have the ability to reduce the complexity of color changes. As a result, in color picture segmentation, this element is utilized to remove shades, reflection, glare, and other light-related concerns.

To overcome these concerns, we created a module that sequentially applied certain picture pre-processing methods. This module performed the following tasks in sequence:

1. Enter the leaf segmented RGB picture in the module

2. Transforms this to HSI

3. Picks the Hue element

4. Applies histogram equalization to Hue

5. finally, transforms the Hue equalized image back to RGB.

To improve the contrast of the Hue picture, histogram equalization is performed on the Hue element. Figure 4.8 shows the result of the transformation of a leaf segmented picture into a Hue Equalized RGB picture by the developed module. The triangle thresholding approach [103] uses the output of this module as an input. Triangle thresholding process is given in Figure 4.7. Flow chart of tringle thresholding is shown in Figure 4.10.

By using threshold binary image is created. When the object pixels produce a weak peak, this approach comes in handy. Figure 4.9 shows the binary picture created by triangle thresholding. This picture contains a black background with a black infected zone.

Triangle thresholding process

Input: RGB image

Output: Computed threshold to create binary image for input

Method ( )

1. Hue Equalized RGB image is first converted in a grayscale

2. Histogram is constructed

3. A line is drawn between the histogram's highest and lowest values.

4. For each value of brightness level L from L = Lmin to L = Lmax, the separation between the line and the histogram hist[L] is determined.

(Here Lmin represents the brightness level on X-axis corresponding to histogram's lowest value (lowest value that is significantly more than 0) and Lmax represents the brightness level on X-axis corresponding to the histogram's highest value.)

5. Separation is computed as Euclidean distance between the line and hist[L].

6. The brightness Level L that corresponds to the maximum separation between hist[L] and the line is chosen as the threshold value.

Figure 4.7 Triangle thresholding Process [103]

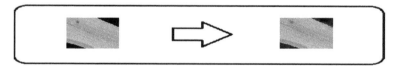

Figure 4.8 Hue Equalized RGB image from Segmented image

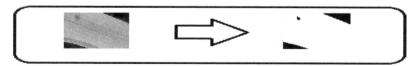

Figure 4.9 Creation of Binary picture by using triangle thresholding process [103]

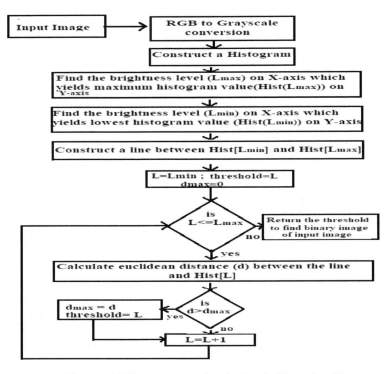

Figure 4.10 Flow chart of triangle thresholding algorithm

4.3.3.4 Estimation of infection severity and partitioning of collected brown spot class

The formula IS= N1 / N2 given in Equ. 4.1 under sub-section 4.3.3.1 is used to calculate severity. Calculating the white pixels count in the binary mask formed by otsu's approach (Figure 4.5) yields the total pixels count in the entire leaf area (N2). Eq. 4.2 is utilized to compute the pixels count in the diseased area (N1) using the binary picture shown in Figure 4.9.

$$(N1) = N_{tb} - N_{ob} \qquad\qquad (4.2)$$

Where N_{tb} denotes the black pixels count in a picture generated by triangle thresholding (Figure 4.9) and N_{ob} is the black pixels count in a binary mask created by Otsu's approach (Figure 4.5).

After the computation of IS for the supplied brown spot leaf picture, it is classified into one of the two categories: ESBS and DSBS. We've set the severity threshold at 0.01 to classify the brown spot illness into one of the two categories (ESBS and DSBS). The following rule is used to categorise the input sample:

For the input brown spot picture

if (IS<= 0.01)

        then keep input picture in ESBS class.

  Otherwise, keep input picture in the DSBS class

Brown spot detection at initial stage means ability to recognise the tiny spots in sample leaf picture (tiny infected areas). Therefore, we attempt to maintain the severity threshold as low as possible for brown spot identification at initial stage. We conducted multiple tests with different alternative criteria less than 1% and found that nearly all photos of acquired brown spot dataset were classified as developed stage brown spot in these circumstances. As a result, we decided on a severity threshold of 1%.

4.3.4 Extraction of Features and Disease detection

CNN has been acknowledged as a significant system for accomplishing image categorization and image identification works in a variety of DIP and computer vision applications. In this chapter, we present a FCNN structure for extracting significant characteristics from input photos automatically.

INPUT: Brown spot diseased dataset
OUTPUT: Early-stage brown spot (ESBS) class and Developed stage brown spot(DSBS)
Start ()
1. Perform first segmentation to get leaf region from the acquired image
      1.1 Resize the image
      1.2 Create Gray-scale image for acquired RGB image
      1.3 Create a binary mask using Otsu's global thresholding method
      1.4 Multiply original RGB image with the binary mask to get leaf region
      1.5 Compute number of pixels for whole leaf region
2. Perform second segmentation on segmented leaf region achieved in step 1 to get infected regions.
      2.1 Create HSI image for segmented leaf region
      2.2 Apply Hue equalization and convert Hue equalized image into RGB
      2.2 Apply Triangle thresholding on Hue equalized RGB image to get segmentation of infected regions
      2.4 Compute number of pixels for infected regions
3. Estimate the infection severity
      3.1 Calculate infection severity using:

Infection Severity= Number of pixels in infected region(N1) / Number of pixels in whole leaf region(N2)

4. Create a new dataset
      4.1 If (IS <= .01)
            then assign input brown spot image to a new Early-stage brown spot class
            otherwise, assign input brown spot image to a new Developed stage brown spot class
5. Repeat the steps from 1 to 4 for each and every image of acquired brown spot diseased dataset

Figure 4.11 Algorithm 1(Infection severity calculation and dataset partition)

The goal of employing the CNN model is to take benefits of it's amazing object identification and categorization learning skills. The model is trained using ESBS, DSBS, and healthy rice leaves classes. One input layer, several combinations of CL and PL combined in a pipelined form, and the FC layers placed as the final layer are the fundamental units of fully connected CNN.

The CL is an essential component of the network that is accountable for learning of the features. The input layer, a succession of CL with ReLU and PL, and FC layers are all used to process each input sample. Each CL uses stride and a 2-dimensional filter to conduct convolution on the input picture to calculate the feature map. During computation of the feature map, the stride is the pixels count necessary to move the filter across the input matrix at a time. A 2-dimensional features map is produced by sliding the filter across the input matrix from left side to right side and from top of matrix to bottom of matrix. Each kernel gets its own feature map.

If the dimension of the input picture matrix is M*N*d and the dimension of the filter matrix is m*n*d, the convolution process produces a features map of dimension (M-m+1) *(N-n+1) *1. The Eq. (3.1) [56] (Specified in chapter 3) is used to calculate the CL's output.

Between the CL and PL, a ReLU layer (RL) is employed. In the outcome of CL, RL induces non-linearity. The negative values of the output matrix produced by convolution operation are set to zero by the ReLU layer while leaving the other values unchanged. ReLU operation is specified in Eq. (3.2) which is illustrated in chapter 3.

The PL is utilized to pool the attributes in the features map created by the ReLU layer. The PL is applied to decrease the dimension of the features map and, as a result, it reduces the number of relevant characteristics needed to categorize illnesses.

In the CNN architecture, we employed four CL units. Each CL unit is comprised of one CL, followed by one BNL, then ReLU, and finally one Max Pool Layer. These CL units worked as hidden layers in the architecture of the network. The first CL applies eight filters (kernels) of 9*9*3 dimension to each resized picture of size 64*64*3. Convolution operation is performed by choosing the value of stride as 1 pixel. The convolution operation of first CL produced the output matrix of dimension 64*64*8. The input channel is then normalised over a specific mini-batch size using BNL. The BNL helps in the speeding up of the learning process while also providing regularisation to prevent network overfitting.

BNL's output is passed on to RL. By performing the basic mathematics described in Eq. 3.2, RL provides non-linear activation. MPL with a pool dimension of 2*2 receives the outcome of RL. MPL selects the highest value from a 2*2 region of the input feature map. It produces 8 features maps of dimension 32*32 when the max-pooling procedure is completed.

The second CL applies 16 filters (kernels) each of 6*6*8 dimension to features map of size 32*32*8 obtained from previous MPL. Convolution operation is performed by choosing the value of stride as 1 pixel. The convolution operation of second CL produced the output matrix of dimension 32*32*16. The output of CL goes through BNL and RL, and finally MPL with a pool dimension of 2*2 is applied on outcome of RL. MPL selects the highest value from a 2*2 region of the input feature map. It produces 16 features maps of dimension 16*16 (output matrix 16*16*16) when the max-pooling procedure is completed.

The third CL applies 32 filters (kernels) each of 3*3*16 dimension to features map of size 16*16*16 obtained from previous MPL. Convolution operation is performed by choosing the value of stride as 1 pixel. The convolution operation of second CL produced the output matrix of dimension 16*16*32. The output of CL goes through BNL and RL, and finally MPL with a pool dimension of 2*2 is applied on outcome of RL. MPL selects the highest value from a 2*2 region of the input feature map. It produces 32 features maps each of dimension 8*8 (output matrix 8*8*32) when the max-pooling procedure is completed.

The fourth CL applies 64 filters (kernels) each of 3*3*32 dimension to features map of size 8*8*32 obtained from previous MPL. Convolution operation is performed by choosing the value of stride as 1 pixel. The convolution operation of second CL produced the output matrix of dimension 8*8*64. The output of CL goes through BNL and RL, and finally, it produced 64 feature maps each of dimension 8*8. Max pooling operation is not used with fourth CL.

Then, as a classification model, 3 FC layers succeeded by a SoftMax layer categorize the input picture into one of three categories (ESBS, DSBS, and Healthy). For each labeled category, SoftMax activation produces probability. During the learning process of the model, the cross-entropy loss is used as a cost function to update the network's weights.

Probability computation for j^{th} class by SoftMax is given in Eq.4.3.

$$P(v_i) = \frac{e^{v_i}}{\sum_{k=1}^{C} e^{v_k}}$$ (4.3)

Here v_i is the input vector for i^{th} class and C is the number of classes in the multi-class classifier.

Eq.4.4. specifies a formula to compute Cross entropy loss (CE).

$$CE = -\sum_{k=1}^{C} t_k \log(P_k)$$ (4.4)

Here t_k is the truth label and P_k is the probability of kth class computed by the SoftMax function.

The suggested fully connected CNN structure's is depicted in Figure 4.12 on next page.

4.4. Experimental Results and Discussions

This section shows the recommended model's experimental environment and performance assessment. The dataset utilized to provide learning to the model, the software and hardware requirements for the investigation, as well as analysis of results, are all included in this section.

4.4.1. Experimental environment

To conduct the experiment, we used the ESBS, DSBS, and Healthy leaves classes as input data. These 3 categories were created using the Brown spot class partitioning approach applied to the paddy leaf samples database [90] (described in section 4.3.3.4). Figure 4.3 depicts the procedure for creating a new data collection for the model's learning. 3008 photographs of ESBS class, 986 photographs of DSBS class, and 4000 photographs of healthy class make up the new dataset for model's learning. Table.4.1 provides a summary of the obtained dataset.

Name	Layer Type	Activations	Learnables	
imageinput	Input	64x64x3	-	imageinput
conv_1	Convolution Layer	64x64x8	Weights 9x9x3x8 Bias 1x1x8	Conv_1
batchnorm_1	Batch Normalization Layer	64x64x8	Offset 1x1x8 Scale 1x1x8	batchnorm_1
relu_1	ReLU Layer	64x64x8	-	relu_1
maxpool_1	Max Pooling Layer	32x32x8	-	maxpool_1
conv_2	Convolution Layer	32x32x16	Weights 6x6x8x16 Bias 1x1x8	Conv_2
batchnorm_2	Batch Normalization Layer	32x32x16	Offset 1x1x16 Scale 1x1x16	batchnorm_2
relu_2	ReLU Layer	32x32x16	-	relu_2
maxpool_2	Max Pooling Layer	16x16x16	-	maxpool_2
conv_3	Convolution Layer	16x16x32	Weights 3x3x16x32 Bias 1x1x32	Conv_3
batchnorm_3	Batch Normalization Layer	16x16x32	Offset 1x1x32 Scale 1x1x32	batchnorm_3
relu_3	ReLU Layer	16x16x32	-	relu_3
maxpool_3	Max Pooling Layer	8x8x32	-	maxpool_3
conv_4	Convolution Layer	8x8x64	Weights 3x3x32x64 Bias 1x1x64	Conv_4
batchnorm_4	Batch Normalization Layer	8x8x64	Offset 1x1x64 Scale 1x1x64	batchnorm_4
relu_4	ReLU Layer	8x8x64	-	relu_4
Fc	Fully Connected Layer (3 Fc layer)	1x1x3	Weights 3x4096 Bias 3x1	Fc
softmax	Softmax Layer	1x1x3	-	softmax
classoutput	Classification Output	-	-	classoutput

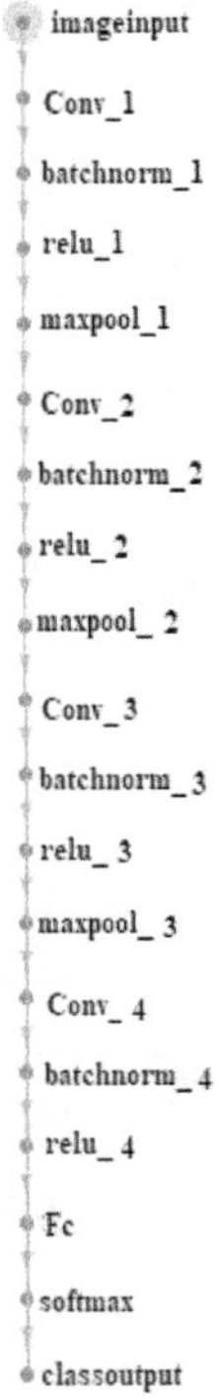

Figure 4.12 Structure of the proposed Fully connected CNN model

The dataset is partitioned into 80:20 partitions, with 80 percent serving as a training dataset and 20 percent serving as a testing dataset to validate the model. Class-wise division of training and validation samples is shown in Table.4.2. All of the experiments are run on a DELL laptop with a Core i5 CPU running at 1.80 GHz. The memory capacity of the above said laptop is four GB DDRAM with 250 GB SSD. This laptop is equipped with Windows 10 OS.

Table 4.1 Summary of created new dataset utilized for model's learning

Leaf Category	Sample's count
Healthy	4,000
ESBS	3,008
DSBS	986

Table 4.2 Class-wise division of training and validation samples

Leaf Category	Training sample's count	Validation sample's count
Healthy	3,200	800
ESBS	2,406	602
DSBS	789	197

4.4.2 Metrics used to evaluate the model's performance

Several assessment parameters are used to evaluate the performance of predictive and classification models [104,105]. In our study, four performance matrices are being used to evaluate the effectiveness of our suggested technique. Here is a brief discussion of these four measures.

1. Accuracy(A): The accuracy of a classification model is calculated as the proportion of correctly categorised samples to the total samples count utilised in classification.

$$A = \frac{\text{Correctly classified samples count}}{\text{Total samples count}}$$

Here Correctly classified samples count is TP+TN, and Total samples count is TP+TN+FP+FN

2. Recall(R): Recall is the proportion of actual positive that is accurately classified or predicted.

$$R = \text{Number of accurately classified positive/Actual Positive}$$

Here Number of accurately classified positive is also known as TP, and Actual Positive = TP +FN

3. Precision(P): Precision is proportion of classified positive that is actually positive.

94

P = Number of accurately classified positive/Classified Positive

Here Number of accurately classified positive is also known as TP, and Classified Positive = TP +FP

4. Overall Accuracy: Overall accuracy is computed as mean of true positives of all classes.

4.4.3 Results and Discussion

The first experiment uses brown spot photos to execute an image processing program in order to determine the severity of the illness. To acquire the ESBS and DSBS from the input brown spot leaves, this experiment utilizes calculated infection severity to split the dataset. The generated dataset includes ESBS and DSBS, as well as healthy leaf samples. The disease recognition model is built in the second experiment. This experiment is carried out by feeding a generated new dataset to the proposed CNN model for the identification of brown spots at a very early stage. In this experiment, we examined the disease recognition results of the suggested system. The classification model is trained and validated using the samples listed in Table 4.2. At a pace of 49 iterations per epoch, we have implemented eight epochs to provide learning to the suggested model. To examine the experimental results, a total of 392 iterations have been experimented. During model validation, the validation frequency is tunned at 5 iterations. The training-validation process is depicted in Figure 4.13. Variation in accuracy against epoch number is shown in Figure 4.13 (a) while variation in loss against epoch number is shown in Figure 4.13 (b). Classification result is analysed using confusion matrix shown in Figure 4.14.

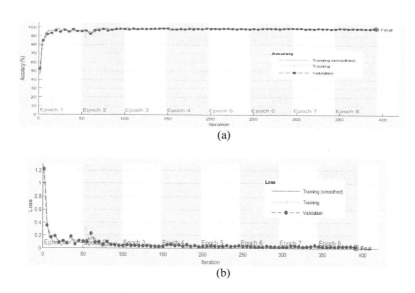

(a)

(b)

Figure 4.13 (a) Training-validation accuracy of suggested model (b) Training-validation Loss-rate of suggested model

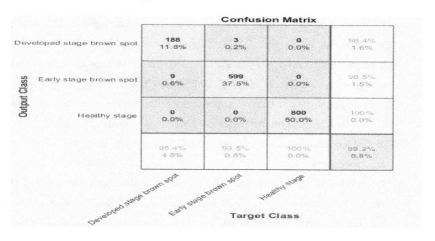

Figure 4.14 Classification results of suggested model using Confusion matrix

96

As we know that all the performance parameters are computed on the basis of "true positive(TP), false positive(FP), true negative(TN) and false negative(FN)" values observed from confusion matrix. For our case, these values are shown in Table 4.3.

Table 4.3 Classification Outcomes

Predicted Classes	(TP)	(FP)	(TN)	(FN)
ESBS	599	9	988	3
DSBS	188	3	1,399	9
Healthy	800	0	799	0

The confusion matrix illustrates the class wise true as well as false classifications done by the suggested model. Class wise precision is shown in the rightmost column and class wise recall is depicted in the bottom row. Overall accuracy of suggested model is depicted in bottom cell of rightmost column.

The created dataset appears to improve the model's learning in such a way that the precisions of ESBS and DSBS classes are obtained as 98.50% and 98.40% respectively whereas a 100 percent precision rate is achieved in healthy class. Class wise recalls (sensitivities) of ESBS, DSBS, and Healthy classes are 99.50%, 95.40%, and 100% respectively. Class wise performance metrices of suggested model is shown in Figure 4.15. Only three cases of Early-stage brown-spot(ESBS) were falsely labeled as developed-stage brown-spot(DSBS) among 608samples, while 9 cases of developed-stage brown spot(DSBS) were incorrectly classified as ESBS out of 201samples. It is observed that our suggested model is both accurate and efficient. The model's training takes only 20 minutes and 17 seconds. The suggested technique achieves an overall accuracy of 99.20 percent, according to the results analysis.

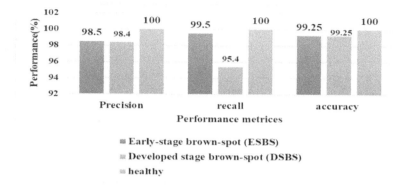

Figure 4.15 Class wise performance parameters

4.4.4 Comparison of accuracy with the related works

We compared the accuracy of our proposed system to the accuracy of other related previous works that classified illnesses based on morphology, size, and color aspects of the infected area from leaf pictures. For automated feature extraction and illness classification, all of the previous models studied here utilised deep CNN architecture. To find the infected regions in the plant leaf, the majority of the examined strategies used image segmentation. In most cases, infection identification and severity calculation were handled independently in other publications.

Our method, on the other hand, integrates illness detection and severity computation into a single unit. The proposed approach has the ability to warn farmers regarding brown spot infection at an initial point. Table 4.4 shows that the methodology presented in this article outperforms the other related methods. Only model suggested by Upadhyay and Kumar (2022) [7] surpasses the suggested technique by a little margin (0.5 percent accuracy), but it is unable to distinguish between the initial and advanced stages of the disease as the suggested system does.

Table 4.4 Comparative analysis

S.No.	Publications	Approaches	Crops	Results
1	Junde Chen et. al. (2020) [4]	Transfer learning approach using VGGNet and Inception pretrained CNN architectures, Image segmentation	Paddy	92.00 percent accurate
2	Sanjay et al. (2020) [64]	A 34-layer RNN model	Paddy	95.83 percent accurate
3	Santosh et al. (2021) [7]	Deep CNN model	Paddy	99.10 percent accurate
4	Santosh et al. (2021) [7]	Deep CNN model with Otsu's method for background removal	Paddy	99.70 percent accurate
5	Upadhyay & Kumar [106] 2021	Proposed Deep CNN architecture for disease identification and categorization, Two-phase image segmentation for severity estimation	Paddy	99.20 percent accurate

4.5 Concluding remarks

The suggested approach is capable of handling massive data sets and automatically extracting the features. The suggested system's strength is its capacity to detect sickness at an early stage. Early detection of brown spots may help farmers to take preventative steps well ahead of time. The usage of insecticides can be decreased if the disease is detected early enough. Controlled application of insecticide not only cuts costs but also minimizes pollution. The suggested system can be used to estimate severity of infection of plant diseases. The suggested technique acts well, with an accuracy of 99.20 percent, according to the results analysis.

CHAPTER 5

TRANSFER LEARNING APPROACH FOR PLANT DISEASE DIAGNOSIS IN PADDY CROPS WITH SMALL DATASET AND COMPLEX IMAGE BACKGROUND

From the discussion of previous chapters, it is very clear that rice is one of the important and preferable grains among agricultural crops but it is susceptible to various viral, bacterial and fungal diseases. In previous chapters we have implemented DCNN model to diagnose such diseases. But many times, the lack of plant leaf picture datasets that can portray the wide range of symptoms and circumstances of features observed in reality is the main problem in using Deep CNN to automatically identify crop diseases. In this chapter, we have discussed about a proposed transfer learning model which can deal these issues effectively. Transfer learning model learns the significant features so deeply and nicely that it gives promising result even for unprocessed input data.

5.1 Introduction

To overcome the issue related to large dataset availability, we apply transfer learning approach and to provide varieties in visual appearance of symptom, we apply image augmentation techniques. These both approaches are applied to build effective disease classification model for Rice crop using InceptionV3 CNN architecture.

5.1.1 Motivation

By the way, many automatic and computerized methods have been developed to diagnose paddy diseases. But most of them are unable to give effective results for small dataset with complex background images. Sometimes it is very difficult to get a large image data set available to provide learning to a deep learning model. Even if a large dataset is available, the deep learning model memorizes the image features due to the lack of variety in the visual appearance of the disease symptoms. These issues cause problem of overfitting. Therefore, there is always search for the techniques, which reduce the problem of overfitting even with small dataset in hand.

5.1.2 Research Objectives

1. To develop a model, which can obtain discriminating features automatically from the leaf images with complex background from small rice leaf dataset.

2. To develop a transfer learning model, which can recognize and classify the 5 types of deadly rice diseases with higher accuracy.

3. To analyze the classification result.

5.1.3 Organization of Chapter

Remaining of this chapter comprise of the following sections:

Section 2 In this section some related works are discussed.

Section 3 This section discusses methods and materials used in "Transfer Learning Approach for Plant Disease Diagnosis in Paddy Crops with Small Dataset and Complex Image Background".

Section 4 This section discusses experimental results and discussions of the proposed model.

Section 5 In this section conclusion of the complete chapter's work is discussed.

5.2 Related Methods

Shrivastava et al. (2019) [107] used TL approach in their study. In their research, they looked at 3 different kinds of paddy leaf infections. Pre-trained CNN model was utilized as features extractor using transfer learning (TL) approach. SVM was used as classifier. The suggested TL approach was found to be 91.37 percent accurate.

Pre-trained Deep CNN models were employed by Hassan et al. (2021) [108] to recognize diseases in plants. They have used the transfer learning (TL) approach to propose a method to recognize the diseases. Pre-trained CNN-based TL models were trained and verified using 53,407 leaf pictures from the PlantVillage database. They

101

used 4 different pre-trained CNN architecture namely InceptionResnetV2, MobileNetV2, InceptionV3, and EfficientNetB0 to develop transfer learning models. EfficientNetB0 beat the other three models, with excellent accuracy of 99.56 percent.

Patil et al. (2021) [109] suggested a deep CNN-based crop disease identification and crop recommender system. For the disease identification system, they have developed 2 models, the first one was a simple deep convolution model and the other was a pre-trained VGG-16-based transfer learning model. A Content-based filtering approach was used to recommend suitable crops. In performance assessment, the VGG-16-based model was found more accurate than simple CNN with a validation accuracy of 97.53 percent.

To diagnose leaves infection in paddy crops, Acharya et al. (2020) [110] used five pre-trained convolution neural networks "ResNet, GoogLeNet, ResNeXt, Wide ResNet, and ShuffleNet" to implement ensemble learning. They acquired images of 3 kinds of leaves. These 3 types of leaves represented 3 types of diseases; 'Brown-spot, BLB, and Blast'. The proposed method has a 95.54 percent accuracy rate.

From the discussion of above transfer learning methods, it is clear that TL models gives higher accuracy.

5.3. Methods And Materials

To diagnose paddy plant illnesses and improve classification, we used the transfer learning strategy with pre-trained DCNN architecture. In this section, we present cutting -edge methods and materials utilized for our study.

5.3.1 Base Methods

In this section, we have discussed about basic components of CNN. Further, structure of InceptionV3 model is discussed. InceptionV3 is a pretrained CNN model, that acts as backbones of the proposed work.

5.3.1.1 CNN

In the last few decades, CNN has proved to be a breakthrough in the domain pattern recognition and computer vision. Nowadays Deep learning, particularly CNN is becoming very popular among researchers because of its accurate classification and effective Learning ability. CNN is a feed-forward NN that is widely used in image recognition. CNN has several hidden layers that have the potential to extract the relevant discriminating features even from complex problems.

The beauty of CNN is that it works well for a very large number of labelled images and effectively processes each and every portion in the images to extract the characterizing features. A typical CNN contains several hidden layers, an input layer, and output layer. CNN accepts the input data especially images as a multidimensional array. Hidden layers contain multiple basic blocks consisting of convolution and pooling layers. These blocks are connected in a sequential manner one after another. The architecture of CNN always performs two types of basic operations namely convolution and pooling operations.

1. Convolution layer (CL): Convolution operation plays an important role to extract feature maps from input image samples. The convolution operation is used to convolved one feature matrix with many different sized filter matrices to get many feature maps (feature matrices). Convolution operation is shown in Figure 5.1 with help of an example.

2. Batch Normalization Layer (BNL): BNL is used to normalise the input channel by re-centering and re-scaling across a particular mini-batch size. Re-centering and re-scaling are performed by computing means and standard deviation across a mini-batch size.

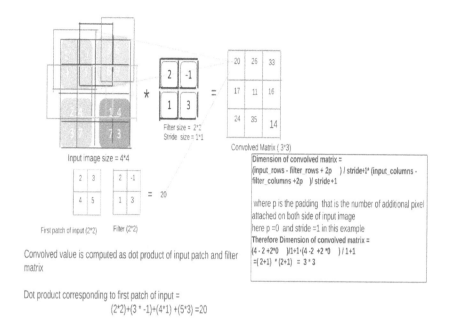

Figure 5.1 Convolution Operation

The BNL assists in accelerating the learning process while simultaneously ensuring network regularisation to avoid overfitting. Batch normalization operation can be applied before or after activation layer. Batch_Norm operation uses batch_ wise mean and variance of input samples. Batch wise mean is calculated by using Eq. (5.1). Batch wise variance is calculated by using Eq. (5.2). Batch normalization computation is shown in Eq. 5.3.

$$mean = \frac{1}{n}\sum_{j=1}^{n} z_j{}^{(i)} \qquad (5.1)$$

$$variance = \frac{1}{n}\sum_{j=1}^{n}(z_j^{(i)} - mean)^2 \qquad (5.2)$$

$$Batch_{Norm} = \frac{Z^{(i)} - mean}{\sqrt{variance + \epsilon}} \qquad (5.3)$$

Where mean, variance and Batch_Norm are the dimension wise computation along a mini-batch. These computations are performed for all input dimensions. Here, n is the size of mini-batch, Z is the d-dimensional input data, $z_j^{(i)}$ is the value of i-th dimension in j-th input data along a mini-batch, $Z^{(i)}$ is the value of i-th dimension of an input.

3. Relu Layers (RL): After the Convolution, the ReLU layer is utilized to convert all negative values of the convolved feature maps to zero. ReLU is recommended as an activation function because of its ability to quickly converge. ReLU operation is shown in figure 5.2.

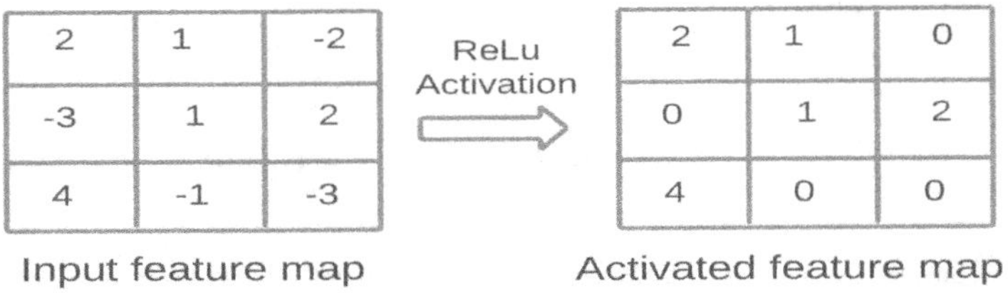

2	1	-2
-3	1	2
4	-1	-3

ReLu
Activation

2	1	0
0	1	2
4	0	0

Input feature map   Activated feature map

Figure 5.2 Relu Activation

4. Pooling Layers (PL): A Pooling Layer is usually applied after a ReLu Layer. This layer's major goal is to lower the dimension of the convolved feature map in order to decrease the computational complexity. Generally, pooling means a small area, therefore a small area is taken of the input matrix and the average value is computed for all cells present in that area in case of average pooling. In the case of max pooling, the greatest value is selected among all cells present in that small chosen pool(area). when pooling is performed on an image, only summarised value (average or max) is taken over all of the present values. Max pooling operation is shown in figure 5.3.

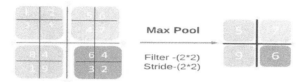

Figure 5.3 Max Pooling operation

5. Fully connected layers (FC)

The CNN's last layer is made up of FC layers (flatten layers) along with a Softmax layer that assign the input picture into any one of the pre-defined categories. A FC is a feed-forward NN that is employed to complete the classification operation. For each labeled category, SoftMax activation produces probability.

5.3.1.2 InceptionV3

The easiest technique to enhance the capabilities of DNN is to raise the breadth and depth of the networks. However, as the breadth and depth of the network grow, it includes more parameters and consumes more computational resources. To address these issues, Szegedy et al. (2016) [111] first incorporated the Inception module into the GoogLeNet architecture, and it won the ImageNet ILSVRC challenge competition with an outstanding performance.

The design of InceptionV3 is divided into two parts: the first is a deep convolutional structure with numerous inception modules to retrieve essential features, and the second is an FC network with SoftMax function at the end to implement classification. The primary objective of this method was to increase efficiency and construct a deeper network to detect complicated attributes from input photos. In the inception modules, CLs with variable kernel sizes (1*1, 1*3, 3*1, 3*3) are executed in parallel, and the outputs are merged before being transmitted to the next layer. Figure 5.4 depicts the architecture of InceptionV3.

106

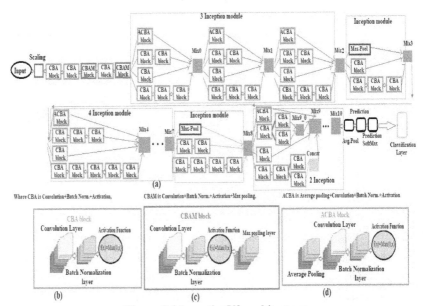

Figure 5.4 InceptionV3 architecture

We updated the native InceptionV3 architecture's last three layers (out of 316 layers) to transfer the learned weights of the pre-trained model to our model dealing with our particular dataset. During fine-tuning, the starting layers of the native InceptionV3 model are locked, and only the last three layers are customized to meet our requirements. Figure 5.10 depicts the customization of layers.

5.3.2 Proposed Work

This section covers the complete process of developing a disease classification and diagnostic model. Figure 5.5 depicts the flow diagram of the proposed system.

5.3.2.1 Image samples collection

We used the rice diseased dataset [113] to get 2,550 photo of rice leaves in 5 categories to provide learning to suggested approach. Each kind of disease consists of 510 image samples. Figure 5.6 shows 5 disease categories on the x-axis and respective image sample counts on the y-axis. Infection symptoms, causing organism and sample images of all 5 diseases are shown in Figure 5.7.

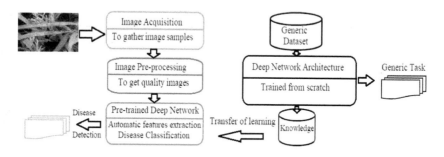

Figure 5.5 Flow diagram of Suggested method

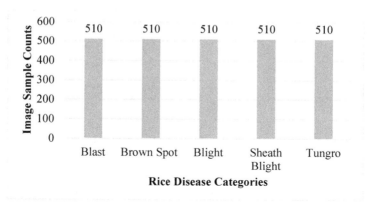

Rice Disease Categories

Figure 5.6 Description of Data set

5.3.2.2 Pre-processing of images

Pre-processing is a crucial step in DIP to produce high-quality photos that meet our needs. Resizing, Contrast stretching, and augmentation are the 3 main preprocessing methods employed in this study. The resizing method is used to create a resized picture with the required input size of 227*227 for InceptionV3.

Disease	Symptoms	Causing Pathogen	Sample Image
Brown Spot	The disease manifests itself as circular to oval spots with dark brown spots	Caused by pathogen: Drechslera oryzae	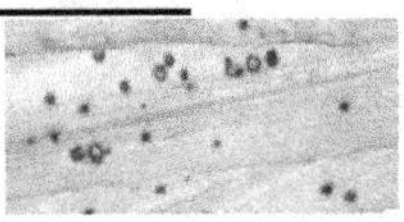
Blast	Oval or spindle-shaped lesions with an ashy greyish centre and a brown border are common.	Caused by fungus: Pyricularia oryzae	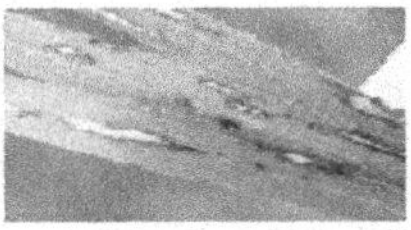
Blight	Symptoms include elongated sores on the leaf tip that are a few inches long. initially white color taht turns to yellow	Caused by bacterium: Xanthomonas oryzae	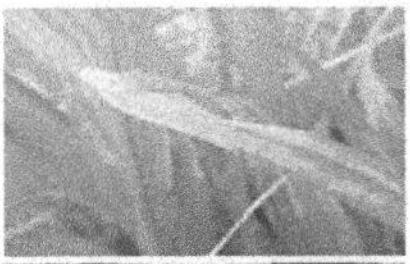
Sheath Blight	Grayish-green-colored lesions are appeared on the leaf sheath. Adjacent infected regions frequently converge, damaging the stem and forcing it to fall and die.	Caused by fungus: Rhizoctonia solani	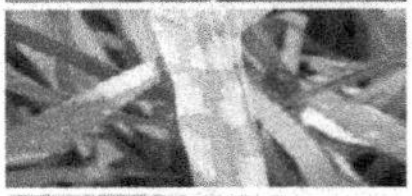
Tungro	Symptoms include empty or partially filled seeds, discolored lesions, slower development, and fewer tillers.	Mixture of two viruses (RTBV and RTSV)	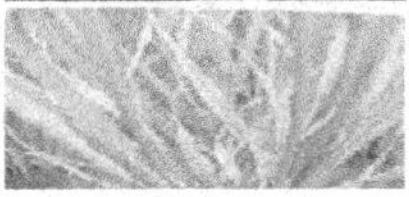

Figure 5.7 Description of dataset's diseases

Contrast stretching operation is applied after resizing the input images. Conversion of RGB photographs to a format that includes luminance information is the first step required to apply the contrast stretching. As a consequence, we transformed resized sample to L*a*b* format. The contrast is adjusted using the luminosity element L*. The luminance is adjusted to vary the pixel intensity while keeping the original colour. The global contrast enhancement of the L component is calculated using Eq.5.4.

$$L_{new}(x,y) = \left(\frac{L_{old}(x,y) - L_{Low}}{L_{High} - L_{Low}}\right) \times 100 \qquad (5.4)$$

Here, $L_{new}(x,y)$ is the new contrast increased luminosity of the pixel (x, y), $L_{old}(x,y)$ is the old luminosity value, L_{High} is the highest luminosity level of the input sample, and L_{Low} is lowest Luminosity level of the input sample.

After the contrast has been adjusted, the image is converted back to RGB format. Transformation of input image to contrast stretched image is shown in figure 5.8.

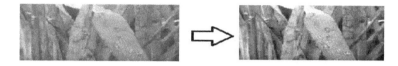

Figure 5.8 Transformation of input image to contrast stretched image

The augmentation method is used to increase the visual diversity of input samples. In this study, the augmentation process includes operations such as reflection, translation, and scaling. Augmented image samples are shown in Figure 5.9. Here, reflection operation randomly reflects the training samples along the y-axis. Translation operation randomly translate the training samples up to 30 pixels vertically and horizontally. Similarly scaling operation scale the training samples 10% vertically and horizontally. Data augmentation prevents the network from being overfit and remembering the exact characteristics of the training pictures.

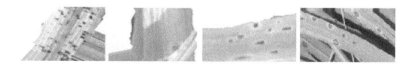

Figure 5.9 Augmented Image Samples

5.3.2.3 Building of suggested model using Transfer Learning (TL)

TL as discussed in Lumini (2019) [112] is a novel learning methodology in which a DCNN model pre-trained on huge dataset is utilized to build a model for another task with specific dataset. In the simple learning process (without TL), the starting weights of the DL model are initialized with random values. Whereas, in transfer learning, the starting weights of the DL model are initialized with the pre-trained model's learned parameters (weights and biases). Thus, transfer learning model utilized learned knowledge of pretrained model to capture the varieties of most significant features from present dataset. In this study, we look into using a InceptionV3 pre-trained on a massive ImageNet [18] database, which is then deployed to the Rice diseased dataset [113]. The basic steps of the TL methodology are given below.

1. Selection of pre-trained DCNN model as foundation:

A InceptionV3 pre-trained DCNN is selected as the base model, and the learned parameters (Biases and weights) of InceptionV3 pre-trained on ImageNet are utilized to assign the initial parameters of the suggested model.

2. Changes to the base model:

Parameters of the initial 313 layers of the base model have been locked. In order to obtain a new customized model that fits on our task, the structure of the rest 3 final layers is changed. Figure 5.10 depicts the changes in the last 3 layers of native InceptionV3 model.

3.Apply finetuning to the customized model: To lower the loss function.

5 categories of leaf pictures from the Rice diseased database are utilized to finetune the customized model.

Layer Number	Native Layers	Modified layers
314	Predictions (1000 fully connected layers)	Predictions (5fully connected layers)
315	Prediction SoftMax (with activation 1x1x1000)	Prediction SoftMax (with activation 1x1x5)
316	Classification Layer (1000 classes)	Classification Layer (5 disease classes)

Figure 5.10 Changes in Native InceptionV3 model

5.3.2.4 Disease Diagnosis and Classification

Three layers of InceptionV3 have been changed to work with the samples we have collected from rice diseased database. In customized InceptionV3 model, the final 1000 FC layers are replaced with 5 FC layers. The SoftMax layer with activation 1*1*1000 has been changed with SoftMax layer with activation 1*1*5. SoftMax activation function is used to determine the classwise probability for the input sample. This probability is used to assess which output class is appropriate for a given input image. finally, classification layer with 1000 classes is changed to the classification layer with 5 classes.

5.4. Implementation and Results

The experimental setting and assessment of performance of the recommended model are shown in this section. This section discusses the disease wise number of samples used to train and test the model, the training-validation process as well as the result analysis.

5.4.1 Experimental Setting

The database of leaf images of rice plant is acquired from the rice diseased dataset. There are five kinds of diseased leaves in this dataset. The dataset is divided into 70:30 partitions, with 70% of the samples acting as training samples and 30% serving as validation samples. The hardware and software utilised in this experiment are the same as those described in chapter 4 under section 4.4.1. Table 5.1 depicts the division of Rice leaf classes into training and testing samples.

Table 5.1 Division of dataset into Training and Testing samples

Disease categories	Training sample counts	Validation Sample counts
Blast	357	153
Brown Spot	357	153
Blight	357	153
Sheath Blight	357	153
Tungro	357	153

5.4.2 Training-validation process

This experiment was conducted by providing pre-processed data samples to the suggested deep CNN model. The proposed model's classification performance was examined on the training and validation dataset (shown in table 5.1). Six epochs were employed, each with 178 iterations. A total of 1,068 iterations were performed to observe the results of the recommended technique. The validation frequency was set to 178 iterations, while the global learning rate was set at 0.0003.

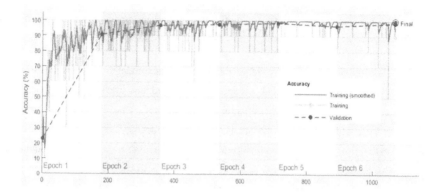

Figure 5.11 Training and Validation Processes of Inception V3

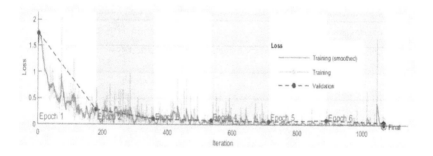

Figure 5.12 Training and validation loss rate of InceptionV3

The validation frequency was set to 178 iterations, while the global learning rate was set at 0.0003. We increased the FC layer's 'BiasLearnRateFactor' and 'WeightLearnRateFactor' values to enable quicker learning in the changed layers than in the fixed layers.

Figure 5.11 depicts the training and validation process. Figure 5.11 shows how the model's accuracy changes as the number of epochs in the training-validation process increase. Figure 5.12 shows how the loss fluctuates as epochs grow. Loss

114

interprets model goodness for validation and training datasets. A better model is one with a lower loss. A confusion matrix is used to demonstrate the model's performance.

5.4.3 Results and Discussion

A confusion matrix is used to demonstrate the model's performance. Figure 5.13 shows the recommended model's correct and incorrect classifications using a confusion matrix. In this confusion matrix, the predicted disease is represented on the y axis, while the actual disease is shown on the x-axis. The confusion matrix (Figure 5.13) illustrates the class wise true as well as false classifications done by the suggested model. Class wise precision is shown in the rightmost column and class wise recall is depicted in the bottom row. The Overall validation accuracy of suggested system is depicted in lowermost cell of rightmost column.

The developed model learned the discriminating characteristics of images in such a good manner that the precisions of all 5 classes are recorded 100% and recall of all 5 classes are recorded 100%. Wrong classification is reduced to zero in all the 5 classes. The Overall validation accuracy of suggested system is obtained as 100 %.

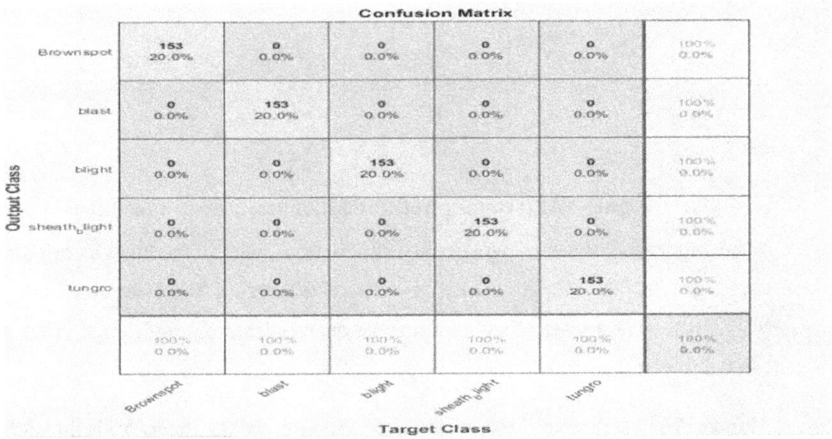

Figure 5.13 Classification results of suggested model using Confusion matrix

115

From the result analysis, it is clear that transfer learning (TL) is able to recognize and classify the diseases with excellent accuracy even with a small dataset and complex background images. Here, the contrast stretching process played a crucial role to enhance the visual appearance of input images. Contrast stretched images are very useful in the extraction of correct and significant features. Further, to achieve variety in visual appearance, an image augmentation process was used. The image augmentation process stops the model to memorize the training features and helps to generalize the learning. Thus, image augmentation reduces the chance of overfitting.

5.4.4 Results comparison of proposed approach with the existing methods

We compared the findings of our proposed model to those of the other relevant existing approaches.

Table 5.2 Comparative analysis of accuracies of proposed model with existing models

Authors	Methods	Plant	Overall Accuracy
Islam et al.,2021[74]	"VGG-19, ResNet-101, Inception-Resnet-V2, and Xception"	Paddy	92.68%
Hassan et al.,2021[108]	MobileNetV2, Inception-ResnetV2, InceptionV3, and EfficientNetB0	14 different plant species	99.56%
Patil et al.,2021[109]	VGG16	------	97.53%
Acharya et al.,2020[110]	Wide ResNet, ResNet, GoogLeNet, ShuffleNet,and ResNeXt	Paddy	95.54%

Proposed approach	InceptionV3	Paddy	100%

All of the approaches compared here used photos of plant leaf samples to detect plant diseases. For illness detection, all the techniques in this comparison utilized the transfer learning approach. We have compared works of Islam et al. (2021) [74] ("VGG-19, ResNet-101, Inception-Resnet-V2, and Xception",), Hassan et al. (2021) [108] (MobileNetV2, Inception-ResnetV2, InceptionV3, and EfficientNetB0), Patil et al. (2021) [109] (VGG16), and Acharya et al. (2020) [110] (Wide ResNet, ResNet, GoogLeNet, ShuffleNet, and ResNeXt). Our approach performed better than that of compared method with an accuracy of 100%. This comparison is shown in table 5.2.

5.5 Concluding Remarks

The suggested approach is capable of handling data sets consisting of images with complex background and also capable of automatically extracting the features from the input samples. The suggested system's strength is its capacity to detect paddy infection with 100% accuracy even with small dataset in hand.

CHAPTER 6

APPLICATION OF TRANSFER LEARNING APPROACH TO DIAGNOSE 9 KINDS OF DEADLY DISEASES FOUND IN TOMATO CROPS

Tomatoes are the most widely consumed vegetable on the earth, and they can be found in any kitchen, irrespective of geography or religion. Tomatoes and their products are immensely popular all around the world. It may be ingested in a variety of ways. After potato and sweet potato, tomato is the third most often grown crop. India is the world's second-largest producer of tomatoes. However, the tomato crop's quality and production are suffering as a result of several infections.

6.1 Introduction

In a country like India, where farming sustains the bulk of the people, detection of infection symptoms of plant diseases becomes very essential. Plant disease identification that is more accurate and faster may help to reduce the impact. The precision and accuracy of plant pathogen recognition systems may be increased with enormous gains and breakthroughs in DL. The objective of this research is to identify leaf diseases in tomato plants and to prevent the economic losses caused by them.

6.1.1 Motivation

Tomato diseases are becoming increasingly difficult to detect using the usual method of human eye inspection. Traditional techniques rely mostly on manuals and specialists' experience as discussed by Singh and Mishra (2017) [29], but the majority of them are labour-intensive, expensive, and time-consuming, as well as they face problems to pinpoint precisely Phung et al. (2018) [93]. As a result, a quick and exact approach to diagnosing tomato diseases is vital for the commercial and environmental well-being of agriculture.

6.1.2 Research Objectives

3. To develop a model, which can obtain discriminating features automatically from the images of tomato leaf samples.

4. To develop a model, which can recognize and classify the 9 types of deadly tomato diseases.

5. To analyze the classification result.

6.1.3 Organization of the Chapter

This Chapter comprise of the following sections:

Section 2 In this section some related works are discussed.

Section 3 This section discusses dataset and methods used in proposed transfer learning model for diagnosis of tomato diseases.

Section 4 This section discusses results analysis and comparative analysis of the proposed model.

Section 5 In this section conclusion of the complete chapter's work is discussed.

6.2 Related Work

Using deep convolution architecture along with Otsu's thresholding, Upadhyay and Kumar (2022) [7] developed a unique approach for diagnosing paddy illnesses. The leaf component was segmented from the obtained input pictures using Otsu's thresholding approach. The recommended CNN model with 4 CL, 3 MPL and four FC layers was fed with segmented pictures to detect and categorise the three categories of rice illnesses. The accuracy of the result analysis was 99.7%.

Agarwal et al. (2020) [57] created a CNN-based model to diagnose illnesses in tomato leaves in their study. Total 3 CL and 3 MPL were utilized in the suggested network, each having a different filter count. They used the tomato leaves image samples from the PlantVillage dataset for this experiment. Total 9 illness categories and one healthy class are in the collection. Since the pictures inside the different categories are unbalanced, image augmentation strategies were used to balance the pictures within the class. The model's validation accuracy ranges from 76 percent to 100 percent for the different categories, according to the result analysis. Furthermore, the model's average validation accuracy was 91.2 percent.

CNN faces several obstacles, such as power and computational load, when it comes to being employed in mobile phones and embedded devices, despite its remarkable improvements in computer vision applications. In this paper, Elhassouny et al. (2019) [114] offered a tomato diseases diagnosis strategy for smartphones that is based on deep CNN. To create this application, they used the MobileNet CNN model, which can distinguish the ten most frequent kinds of tomato leaf infections. 7176 photos of tomato leaves were used to construct the suggested model. These images were acquired from tomato leaf dataset. The suggested model has performed 90.30 percent accurate classification in result validation.

Using transfer learning and feature concatenation, the Al-Gaashani et al. (2022) [115] offered a technique for classifying diseases found in tomato leaves. The authors extracted features from NASNetMobile and MobileNetV2 using pre-trained learned weights, then used kernel principal component analysis to concatenate and minimize the dimensions of extracted features. They then integrate these characteristics into a traditional learning system. The findings of the experiments support the use of concatenated features to enhance the effectiveness of the suggested model. "Multinomial logistic regression, support vector machine, and random forest" were the 3 most common classical ML classifiers assessed by the authors. Results analysis showed that multinomial logistic regression obtained the greatest accuracy of 97 percent.

Zaki et al. (2020) [116] applied transfer learning to diagnose and categorise leaf infections in tomato plants using the MobileNetV2 pre-trained model. Suggested model is trained on 4,671 photos acquired from plant-village-dataset. According to the results analysis the presented model has a 90% accuracy in identifying the infections.

6.3. Methods And Materials

To diagnose tomato plant illnesses and improve classification, we used the transfer learning strategy with pre-trained DCNN architecture. In this section, we present cutting -edge methods and materials utilized for our study.

6.3.1 Base Methods

In this section, we have discussed about structure of SqueezeNet model. SqueezeNet is a pretrained CNN model, that acts as backbones of the proposed work.

6.3.1.1 CNN

CNN is a feed-forward NN that is widely used in image recognition. CNN has several hidden layers that have the potential to extract the relevant discriminating features even from complex problems. Fundamental structure of CNN is depicted in Figure 6.1. Description of CNN with different components is explained in chapter 5 under section 5.3.1.1.

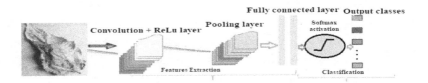

Figure 6.1 Fundamental structure of CNN

6.3.1.2 SqueezeNet

This design was presented by Iandula et al. in 2016 [117]. It is a DCNN that is pre-trained on a massive ImageNet dataset. SqueezeNet employs architectural strategies to minimize the parameter counts, primarily with the use of fire modules, which "squeeze" parameters using convolutions with 1x1 filters.

A total of eighteen deep layers are arranged in SqueezeNet architecture. Nine fire modules are placed between 2 CLs in SqueezeNet. The fire modules have a squeeze CL with 1*1 kernels and an expand layer with two convolutions in parallel with

121

distinct filters of dimensions 1*1 and 3*3 correspondingly. The squeeze layer's outcome is supplied to the expand layer in the fire module. Architecture of squeezeNet is depicted in Figure 6.2.

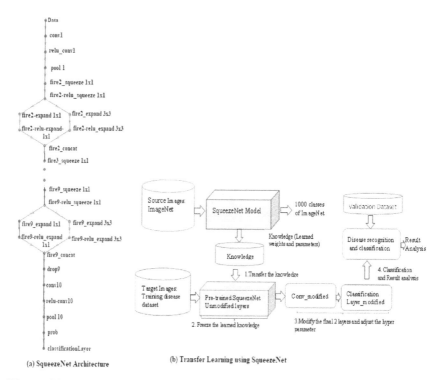

(a) SqueezeNet Architecture

(b) Transfer Learning using SqueezeNet

Figure 6.2 Architecture of SqueezeNet and Transfer learning process using SqueezeNet

Combining this with the fact that SqueezeNet obtains the same performance as AlexNet while having 50 times fewer weights leads us to believe that SqueezeNet may be the best CNN design for this purpose.

6.3.2 Proposed Work

This section covers the entire process of creating a disease diagnosis and categorization model. Figure 6.3 shows a flow diagram of the suggested system.

6.3.2.1 Image samples collection

We used the benchmarked PlantVillage database [118] to get 16012 tomato leaves pictures in ten categories ("9 diseased leaf classes and 1 healthy leaf class") to provide learning to recommended approach. Figure 6.4 shows ten categories on the x-axis and respective image sample counts on the y-axis.

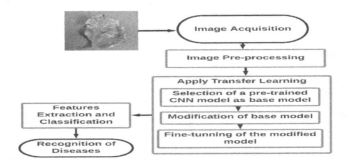

Figure 6.3 Suggested system's flow diagram

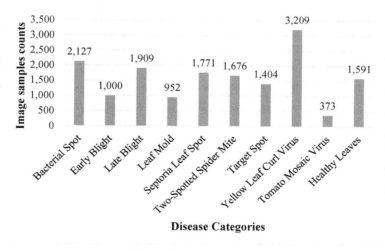

Figure 6.4 Dataset description

Sample images of 9 kinds of diseased leaves and 1 healthy leaf acquired from dataset are depicted in Figure 6.5.

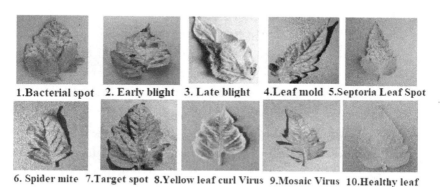

Figure 6.5 Sample images of diseases acquired from dataset [118]

6.3.2.2 Pre-processing of images

Pre-processing is an important step in obtaining quality images as per our requirements. The major preprocessing techniques used in this work are resizing and augmentation. The resizing process is utilized to get resized image of size 227*227, which is the required input size for SqueezeNet. The augmentation process is used to get more visual varieties of input samples. Reflection, translation, scaling, and rotation operations are performed during the augmentation process in this research work.

6.3.2.3 Building of suggested model using TL

TL is a new type of learning strategy in which a model trained for one task is used as the basis for a model for another task. In the usual learning procedure, the Initial parameters of the network were initialized with random values. However, instead of performing learning from the start, the suggested deep network's initial parameters are initialized with the pre-trained model's learned parameters (weights and biases). In this study, we look into using a SqueezeNet pre-trained on a massive ImageNet database, which is then deployed to the PlantVillage database's leaves samples. The primary steps of the transfer learning strategy are as follows.

1. Selection of pre-trained DCNN model as foundation:

A SqueezeNet pre-trained DCNN is selected as the base model, and the learned parameters (Biases and weights) of SqueezeNet pre-trained on ImageNet are utilized to assign the initial parameters of the suggested modified model.

2. Changes to the base model:

Parameters of the initial 63 layers of the base model have been locked. To get a new customized model design, the architecture of the rest 5 final layers is altered by replacing the layers. Table 6.1 depicts the changes in the five layers.

3. Apply finetuning to the customized model:

To lower the loss function, 10 categories of leaf pictures from the Plant Village database are utilized to finetune the customized model.

Table 6.1 Customization of SqueezeNet

Layer Number	Native Layers	Modified layers
64	Predictions convolution2dLayer (1000 convolutions with activation 14x14x1000)	Predictions convolution2dLayer (10 convolutions with activation 14x14x10)
65	Prediction relu_convolution (with activation 14x14x1000)	Prediction relu_convolution (with activation 14x14x10)
66	Prediction average pooling (with activation 1x1x1000)	Prediction average pooling (with activation 1x1x10)
67	Prediction SoftMax (with activation 1x1x1000)	Prediction SoftMax (with activation 1x1x10)
68	Classification Layer (1000 classes)	Classification Layer (10 output classes)

6.3.2.4 Disease Diagnosis and Classification

SqueezeNet has been modified to suit our collected samples. The final learnable CL is substituted by a CL with the same number of kernels as the count of class labels (10 in our database) in the tomato leaf database. To calculate the classwise likelihood for the input sample, the SoftMax layer employs a SoftMax activation function. This likelihood is utilized to determine which output class is acceptable for a particular input picture.

6.4. Experimental Results and Discussions

This section shows the suggested model's experimental environment and performance assessment. The dataset utilized to provide learning to the model, the software and hardware requirements for the investigation, as well as analysis of results, are all included in this section.

6.4.1 Experimental Environment

The dataset with picture of tomato leaves is obtained via PlantVillage database [118]. There are nine categories of sick leaves in this dataset, as well as one category of healthy leaves. On this dataset, we have conducted an experiment using transfer learning strategy. The dataset is partitioned into 70:30 partitions, with 70 percent serving as training samples and 30 percent serving as testing samples to validate the model. The hardware and software used in this experiment is same as specified in chapter 4 under section 4.4.1. Division of Tomato leaf classes into training and testing samples is depicted in Figure 6.6.

6.4.2 Training-validation process

This experiment was carried out by feeding the suggested deep CNN model with pre-processed data samples with 9 kinds of different illnesses. Here, we have evaluated the suggested model's classification performance for acquired tomato leaf samples. The model's training and validation were experimented using the training-validation samples depicted in Figure. We used six epochs, each of which had 373 iterations. To observe the results of suggested approach, a total of 2238 iterations were performed. Training and Validation process are illustrated in figure 6.7. Here, Figure 6.7 depicts how model's accuracy changes with the increment in the number of epochs in training-validation process.

Figure 6.8 illustrates the changes in the loss as the number of epochs increases. For validation and training datasets, Loss interprets model goodness. A model with a smaller loss is a better model. The model's performance is depicted using a confusion matrix. The suggested model's right and wrong classifications are depicted in Figure 6.9 using a confusion matrix. Here, predicted disease is shown along y axis whereas actual disease is shown along x-axis in confusion matrix. The frequency of validation is set at 10 iterations. The learning rate is set at 0.0003.

Categories of tomato diseases	Training sample counts	Validation sample counts	Sample leaf images
Bacterial Spot	1,489	638	
Early Blight	700	300	
Late Blight	1,336	573	
Leaf Mold	666	286	
Septoria Leaf Spot	1,240	531	
Two-Spotted Spider Mite	1,173	503	
Target Spot	983	421	
Yellow Leaf Curl Virus	2,246	963	
Tomato Mosaic Virus	261	112	
Healthy Leaves	1,114	477	

Figure 6.6 Division of Tomato leaf classes into training and testing samples

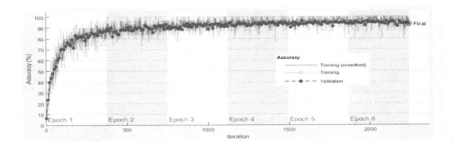

Figure 6.7 Training-validation process of the model

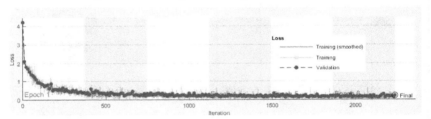

Figure 6.8 Training-validation loss rate of the model

Confusion Matrix

Output Class	Bacterial Spot	Early Blight	Late Blight	Leaf Mold	Septoria Leaf Spot	Two-Spotted Spider Mite	Target Spot	Yellow Leaf Curl Virus	Tomato Mosaic Virus	Healthy Leaves	
Bacterial Spot	612	4	1	0	1	0	0	15	0	0	96.7%
	12.7%	0.1%	0.0%	0.0%	0.0%	0.0%	0.0%	0.3%	0.0%	0.0%	3.3%
Early Blight	1	218	6	0	0	0	0	0	0	0	96.6%
	0.0%	4.5%	0.1%	0.0%	0.0%	0.0%	0.0%	0.0%	0.0%	0.0%	3.1%
Late Blight	2	15	523	0	0	0	0	0	0	0	96.9%
	0.0%	0.3%	10.9%	0.0%	0.0%	0.0%	0.0%	0.0%	0.0%	0.0%	3.1%
Leaf Mold	0	0	0	228	0	1	0	0	0	0	99.6%
	0.0%	0.0%	0.0%	4.7%	0.0%	0.0%	0.0%	0.0%	0.0%	0.0%	0.4%
Septoria Leaf Spot	4	45	31	43	529	0	26	0	1	0	77.9%
	0.1%	0.9%	0.6%	0.9%	11.0%	0.0%	0.5%	0.0%	0.0%	0.0%	22.1%
Two-Spotted Spider Mite	0	1	0	4	0	446	1	2	0	0	98.2%
	0.0%	0.0%	0.0%	0.1%	0.0%	9.3%	0.0%	0.0%	0.0%	0.0%	1.8%
Target Spot	19	13	2	1	0	36	382	0	0	0	84.3%
	0.4%	0.3%	0.0%	0.0%	0.0%	0.7%	8.0%	0.0%	0.0%	0.0%	15.7%
Yellow Leaf Curl Virus	0	2	2	0	0	1	0	945	0	0	99.5%
	0.0%	0.0%	0.0%	0.0%	0.0%	0.0%	0.0%	19.7%	0.0%	0.0%	0.5%
Tomato Mosaic Virus	0	2	0	9	1	9	2	0	111	0	82.8%
	0.0%	0.0%	0.0%	0.2%	0.0%	0.2%	0.0%	0.0%	2.3%	0.0%	17.2%
Healthy Leaves	0	0	8	1	0	10	10	0	0	477	94.3%
	0.0%	0.0%	0.2%	0.0%	0.0%	0.2%	0.2%	0.0%	0.0%	9.9%	5.7%
	95.9%	72.7%	91.3%	79.7%	99.6%	88.7%	90.7%	98.2%	99.1%	100%	93.1%
	4.1%	27.3%	8.7%	20.3%	0.4%	11.3%	9.3%	1.8%	0.9%	0.0%	6.9%

Target Class

Figure 6.9 Classification results of suggested model using Confusion matrix

6.4.3 Results and Discussion

The confusion matrix (Figure 6.9) illustrates the class wise true as well as false classifications done by the suggested model. Class wise precision is shown in the rightmost column and class wise recall is depicted in the bottom row. The Overall validation accuracy of suggested system is depicted in lowermost cell of rightmost column.

The developed model learned the discriminating characteristics of images in such a good manner that the precisions of 6 classes (out of 10) are recorded more than 96% and recall of 5 classes (out of 10) are recorded more than 95%. Wrong classification is reduced to zero in healthy classes. The Overall validation accuracy of suggested system is obtained as 93.10 %. Classwise recall and precision parameters are shown in Fig. 6.11. and Fig. 6.10, respectively.

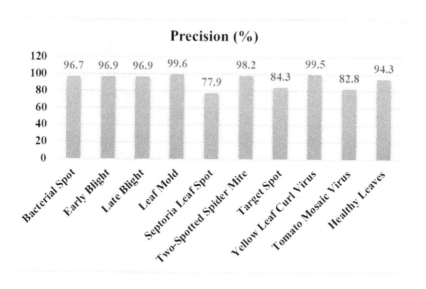

Figure 6.10 Class-wise performance in terms of precision

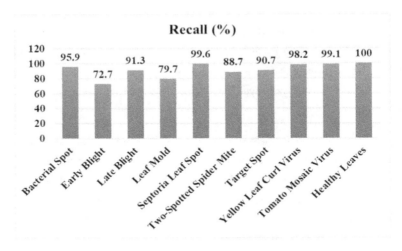

Figure 6.11 Class-wise performance in terms of recall

5.4.4 Results comparison of proposed approach with the existing methods

We compared our technique to three previously published publications in the field. Leaf photos of tomato illnesses were utilized by all compared work for training and testing of the model. Here leaf samples were obtained from the PlantVillage collection. All the methods compared in this analysis used nine illnesses of the same kind. Two of the existing works (Zaki et al., 2020 [116] and Elhassouny and Smarandache, 2019 [114]) used the TL approach to identify 9 deadly diseases, while the other (Agarwal et al., 2020 [57]) used a simple CNN model with three CL, three PL, and two FC layers to identify the infections. Zaki et al. used MobilenetV2 and Elhassouny used MobileNet as base model for transfer learning. Our approach performed better than the compared method in terms of accuracy, which is shown in figure 6.12.

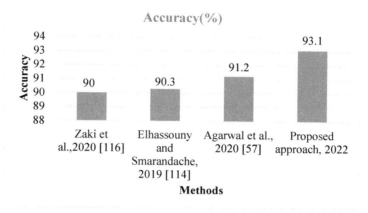

Figure 6.12 Performance comparison with existing method

6.5 Concluding remarks

The suggested approach is capable of handling 9 types of deadly tomato diseases and is capable of automatically extracting the features from input samples. By the way, many automatic and computerized methods have been developed to diagnose tomato diseases. But most of them are unable to handle 9 varieties of diseases. Some of the methods detect same 9 diseases as we have detected, but in these cases our approach performed better with an accuracy of 93.10%.

CHAPTER 7
CONCLUSION & FUTURE WORK

Plant pathogens may have a devastating influence on food safety, as well as a considerable loss in both the quantity and amount of farming goods. Crop Illnesses can potentially prevent grain harvesting completely in extreme circumstances. As a result, in the case of agricultural technology, computerized diagnosis and detection of plant pathogens are widely needed. Many approaches to solving this problem have been offered, with deep learning emerging as the favoured option because of its excellent result. DCNN has recently achieved significant progress in several disciplines related to computer vision, such as outperforming human-level perception, image segmentation, object recognition, and categorization.

The important contributions of the thesis are concluded in this chapter, and some relevant directions for further research are recommended. The thesis concluding remark is discussed in Section 7.1, and Section 7.2 offers proposals for future work related to plant leaf disease detection.

7.1 Conclusion

The first research objective of this thesis is achieved by conducting literature review to identify the research gaps.

Next, we have explored whether a simple fully connected Convolution Neural Network architecture can be designed and utilized to recognize and classify the rice plant illnesses effectively by using images of plant leaf, and whether a background removal technique can be utilised to increase the performance even more.

For exploration, we have developed a simple fully connected CNN for rice illness(pathogen) recognition and classification using leaf images. Number of filters and size of filters in convolution operation are designed in such a good manner that it outperformed the existing methods with an accuracy of 99.1%. We have used large dataset to overcome the problem of overfitting. To boost performance even more, we have applied background removal technique on input images before feeding it into suggested FCNN. Here, background removal technique is implemented using Otsu's global thresholding method. Removal of background from input leaf images, further enhance the classification accuracy with a margin of 0.6%. This way, we have achieved second research objective.

Generally, it has been observed that due to lack of proper knowledge of disease intensity, the farmer is not able to use the pesticide in proper quantity to treat the diseases. The use of pesticide mostly becomes more than necessary, due to which there is not only a loss of money, but also it causes soil and environmental pollution. If disease severity-wise labelled data sets are available, it can be used to develop pesticide recommendation systems. Images with least infection severity can be used to train and validate a DL model to capture the plant diseases at very initial stage. In this thesis, third research objective related to this issue is successfully achieved by introducing an infection severity estimation method based on two phase image segmentation technique to derive new dataset labelled with disease intensity from existing plant disease dataset. First segmentation is performed by Otsu's thresholding approach to obtain leaf part from the input sample. Second segmentation is performed by triangle thresholding method to get infected parts from leaf region. Infection severity computation is done on the basis of infected and non-infected pixels counts present in leaf image samples. This derived dataset played an important role to achieve fourth research objective.

Many times, it has been seen that the plant diseases only become visible when its effect has spread out. Therefore, to reduce the impact of plant diseases, it is not enough to recognize the disease only, but it is necessary to capture the infection at early stage. This observation became the basis of the fourth objective.

To achieve the fourth objective, we have developed a simple fully connected CNN model by using infection severity based derived leaf image dataset to identify the brown spot rice diseases accurately at early stage. The suggested approach performed well with 99.20% accuracy.

The final objective is achieved by developing 2 transfer learning models, one for diagnosis of paddy diseases with small dataset in hand and other for diagnosis of 9 types of deadly tomato diseases. Both the model performed well. Transfer learning model for paddy disease diagnosis achieved 100% accuracy even with small dataset with complex background images. Other transfer learning model for tomato disease diagnosis detect 9 types of tomato diseases with an accuracy of 93.10%. Comparative analysis shown that this accuracy is better than other related method.

7.2 Future Work

Following are the few suggestions for future work.

1. We are primarily focusing on 2 crops diseases namely; paddy diseases and tomato diseases. This work can be extended to cover more crop diseases.
2. This work mainly focuses on leaf of plant to diagnose the plant diseases. Future work could focus on extending the suggested work to diagnose the plant diseases using stems, fruits, and flowers.
3. Our approach assume that one leaf is infected by only one disease. This work can be extended to diagnose the multiple diseases in a single leaf.
4. This work can be applied on real field dataset collected directly from crop fields by IoT system.
5. This study may be extended to include the development of a mobile application for the proposed technique to automatically recognise and monitor a variety of crop diseases using smartphones and tablets.

CPSIA information can be obtained
at www.ICGtesting.com
Printed in the USA
BVHW051539200423
662734BV00011B/313